Soccer Tryouts:

A Step-by-Step Guide on How to Make the Team

Dylan Joseph

Soccer Tryouts:
A Step-by-Step Guide on How to Make the Team

By: Dylan Joseph
© 2020

WAIT!

Wouldn't it be nice to have the steps in this book on an easy one-page checklist for you to make preparing and succeeding in your tryouts even easier? Well, here is your chance!

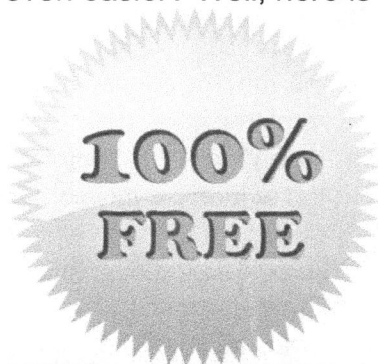

UNDERSTANDSOCCER.COM - TRYOUT CHECKLIST

✓ Before Tryouts Start
- Avoid working out at least two days prior to the start of tryouts.
- Eat a nutritious meal. (i.e. chicken, a fruit, a vegetable, and a grain/carb.)
- Have all your gear? (Ball, cleats, shin guards, socks, etc.)
- Wear the same bright color each day to stand out.
- Bring your medical physical, if needed.
- Apply *sunscreen* if it is a sunny day.
- Bring snacks like a banana or apple if the tryout is several hours.
- Drink a 16 oz. water bottle to make sure that you are hydrated.
- 30 mins prior to start, drink a pre-workout like: *Pure Pump*
     Watermelon Naked Energy   *Garden of Life Energy + Focus*
- Get to the field early (at least 30 mins).
- Remember, the feelings you have right now are feelings of excitement.
- Warm up for at least 10 minutes before the actual tryouts start.

✓ During Tryouts
- Make a great first impression - Shake the coach's hand and introduce yourself.
- Make eye contact, smile, and stand up straight.
- Tryout in the position you want to play.
- Show off your strengths.
- Communicate & direct other people what to do in scrimmages.
- If a coach gives you feedback, implement it immediately.
- Make sure at least 95% of your first touches are attacking touches.
- Outwork others. Hustle, hustle, hustle!
- If you make a mistake, don't sweat it. Recover from it as best you can.
- Drink a 16 oz. bottle of water for every hour of tryouts.

✓ After Tryouts
- Thank the coach & give him or her another strong handshake.
- Stretch.
- Ice any body parts that hurt once you get home.
- Drink a 16 oz. water bottle to help with recovery.
- Take a post workout *whey protein supplement* or drink some milk.

©Understand, LLC

Go to this Link for an **Instant** One-Page Printout:
UnderstandSoccer.com/free-printout

This FREE checklist is simply a thank you for purchasing this book. This one-page checklist will ensure that the knowledge you obtain from this book helps you make the team.

Table of Contents

Dedication

This book is dedicated to all the soccer players, coaches, and parents who are reading this book to improve their knowledge and to strengthen others around them. Whether it be for yourself, your team, or your child, growing to help others and yourself develop is exceptionally noble and speaks volumes to the person you are.

Preface

Tryouts can be one of the scariest things that you do in your life. Knowing that every move you make will be judged by one or more coaches can make a player trying out very nervous. However, with the right tips, tricks, tweaks, and techniques on how to be a top performer in a tryout, you can go into a tryout knowing that you have a ton of confidence and are excited and not nervous to show off your abilities.

The knowledge in this book is only helpful when applied. Therefore, apply it to be sure you can impress the coaches, be recognized as a leader on the field, stand out among all the other players trying out, and feel confident after the tryouts are completed knowing that you have made the team. For any words you are unsure of the meaning, please reference the glossary in the back of the book.

INDIVIDUAL SOCCER PLAYER'S PYRAMID

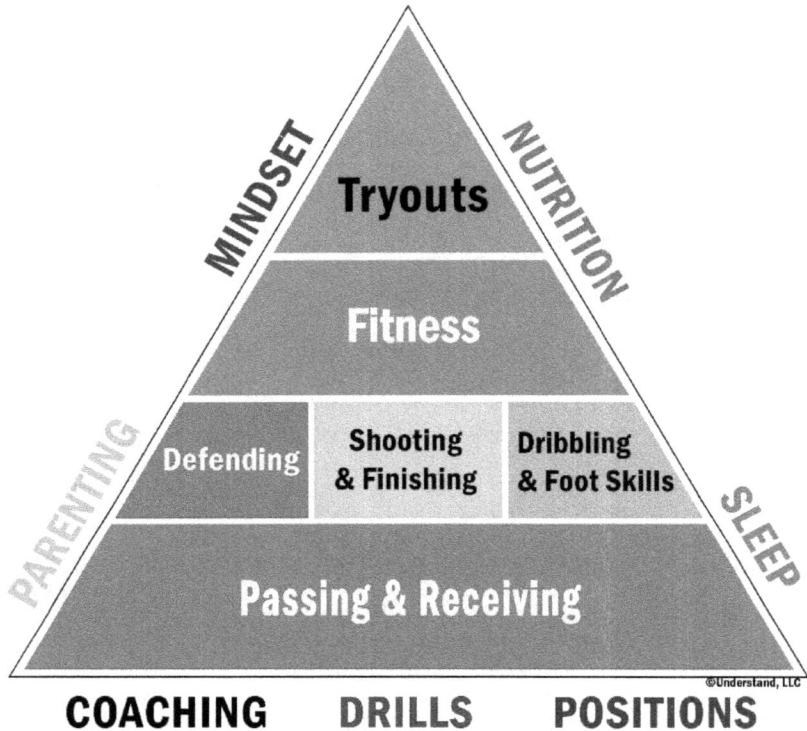

If you are looking to improve your skills, your child's confidence, or your players' abilities, it is essential to understand where this book fits into the bigger picture of developing a soccer player. In the image, the most critical field-specific skills to work on are at the base of the Individual Soccer Player's Pyramid. The pyramid is a quality outline to improve an individual soccer player's game. All the elements in the pyramid and the items surrounding it play a meaningful part in becoming a better player, but certain skills should be read and mastered first before moving on to the others.

You will notice that passing and receiving is at the foundation of the pyramid. This is because if you can receive and make a pass in soccer, then you will be a useful teammate. Even though you may not consistently score, dispossess the other team, or dribble through several opponents, you will still have the fundamental tools needed to play the sport and contribute to your team.

As you move one layer up, you find yourself with a decision to make on how to progress. Specifically, the pyramid is created with you in mind because each soccer player and each soccer position has different needs. Therefore, your choice regarding which path to take first is dictated by the position you play and more importantly, by the position that you want to play. In soccer and life, just because you are in a particular spot, position, or even a job, it does not mean that you have to stay there forever if that is not your choice. However, it is not recommended to refuse playing a position if you are not in the exact role you want. It takes time to develop the skills that will allow you to make a shift from one position to another.

If you want to become a forward, then consider starting your route on the second layer of the pyramid with shooting and finishing. As your abilities to shoot increase, your coach will notice your new finishing skills and will be more likely to move you up the field (if you are not a forward already). Be sure to communicate to the coach that you desire to be moved up the field to a more offensive position, which will increase your chances, as well. If you are already a forward, then dive deep into this topic to ensure you become the leading scorer; first on your team, and then in the entire league. Notice that shooting and finishing is considered less critical than passing and receiving. This is because you have to pass the ball up the field before you can take a shot on net.

Otherwise, you can start by progressing to dribbling & foot skills from passing & receiving because the proper technique is crucial to dribble the ball well. It is often necessary for a soccer player to use a skill to protect the ball from the other team or to advance the ball up the field to place their team in a favorable situation to score. The selection of this route is often taken first by midfielders and occasionally by forwards.

Defending is another option of how you can proceed from passing and receiving. Being able to keep the other team off the scoreboard is not an easy task. Developing a defender's mindset, learning which way to push a forward, understanding how to position your body, knowing when to foul, and using the correct form for headers is critical to a defender on the back line looking to prevent goals.

Finish all three areas in the second layer of the pyramid before progressing up the pyramid. Dribbling and defending the ball (not just shooting) are useful for an attacker; shooting and defending (not just dribbling) are helpful for a midfielder, while shooting and dribbling (not just defending) are helpful for a defender. Having a well-rounded knowledge of the skills needed for the different positions is important for all soccer players. It is especially essential for those soccer players who are looking to change positions in the future. Shooting and finishing, dribbling and foot skills, and defending are oftentimes more beneficial for soccer players to learn first, so focus on these before spending time on the upper areas of the pyramid. In addition, reading about each of these areas will help you to understand what your opponent wants to do.

Once you have improved your skills in the first and second tiers of the pyramid, move up to fitness. It is difficult to go through a passing/dribbling/finishing drill for a few minutes without being out of breath. However, as you practice everything below the fitness category in the pyramid, your fitness and strength will naturally increase. Performing technical drills allows soccer players to increase their fitness naturally. This reduces the need to focus exclusively on running for fitness.

Coming from the perspective of both a soccer player and trainer, I know that constantly focusing on running is not as fulfilling and does not create long-lasting improvements, whereas emphasizing shooting capabilities, foot skills, and defending knowledge creates long-lasting change. Often, coaches who focus on running their players in practice are also coaches who want to improve their team but have limited knowledge of many of the soccer-specific topics that would quickly increase their players' abilities. Not only does fitness in soccer include your endurance; it also addresses your ability to run with agility and speed and to develop strength and power, while using stretching to improve your flexibility. All these tools put together leads to a well-rounded soccer player.

Similar to the tier below it, you should focus on the fitness areas that will help you specifically, while keeping all of the topics in mind. For example, you may be a smaller soccer player who could use some size. In this case, you should emphasize weight training so that you can gain the muscle needed to avoid being pushed off the ball. However, you should still stretch before and after a lifting workout or soccer practice/game to ensure that you stay limber and flexible to recover quickly and avoid injuries.

Maybe you are a soccer player in your 20s, 30s, or 40s. Then, emphasizing your flexibility would do a world of good to ensure you keep playing soccer for many more years. However, doing a few sets of push-ups, pull-ups, squats, lunges, sit-ups, etc. per week will help you maintain or gain a desirable physique.

Furthermore, you could be in the prime of your career in high school, college, or at the pro level, which means that obtaining the speed and endurance needed to run for 90+ minutes is the most essential key to continue pursuing your soccer aspirations.

Finally, we travel to the top of the pyramid, which involves tryouts. Although tryouts occur only 1-2 times per year, they have a huge impact on whether you will make the team or get left out of the lineup. Tryouts can cause intense anxiety if you do not know the keys to make sure that you stand out from your competitors and are very confident from the start.

If you have not read the *Understand Soccer* series book, *Soccer Training*, it is highly recommended that you do to gain the general knowledge of crucial topics within the areas of the pyramid. Picking up a copy of the book will act as a good gauge to see how much you know about each topic, which will help determine if a book later in the series written about a specific subject in the soccer pyramid will be beneficial for you.

The last portion of the pyramid are the areas that surround the pyramid. Though these are not skills and topics that can be addressed by your physical abilities, they each play key roles in rounding out a complete soccer player. For example, having a supportive parent/guardian or two is beneficial for transporting the child to games, providing the equipment needed, the fees for the team, expenses for individual training, and encouragement. Having a quality coach whose teachings and drills help the individual learn how their performance and skills fit into the team's big picture helps a lot too.

Sleeping enough is critical to having enough energy during practices and on game days, in addition to recovering from training and games. Appropriate soccer nutrition will increase a soccer player's energy and endurance, help them achieve the ideal physique, and significantly aid in their recovery.

Understanding soccer positions will help you determine if a specific role is well-suited for your skills. It is important to know that there are additional types of specific positions—not just forwards, midfielders, and defenders. A former or current professional player in the same position as you can provide guidance on the requirements to effectively play that position.

Finally, you must develop a mindset that will leave you unshakable. This mindset will help you prepare for game situations, learn how to deal with other players, and be mentally tough enough to not worry about circumstances that you cannot control, such as the type of field you play on, the officiating, or the weather.

The pyramid is a great visual aid to consider when choosing what areas to focus on next as a soccer player, coach, or parent. However, remember that a team's pyramid may look slightly different based on which tactics the players can handle and which approach the coach decides to use for games. Now that you know where this book plays into the bigger picture, let us begin.

Remember that if there are any words or terms whose meaning you are unsure of; you can feel free to reference the glossary at the back of the book.

If you enjoy this book, please leave a review on Amazon letting me know.

Introduction

Soccer Tryouts was written to ensure you make the team you are trying out for. Personally, I have made several teams in my career that I had no business being on if you just considered only my soccer skills! However, by focusing on showing off my strengths in the tryout and using a few tricks mentioned in this book, I ensured that I stood out from the crowd and was frequently picked by the coaching staff for their soccer teams. Most of the tricks were completely unrelated to being good at soccer—which, at the time, was exactly what I needed because I had still yet to learn many of the skills discussed in the other books in the *Understand Soccer* series.

Granted, I got a lot better over time, and playing with and against kids who were much better than me helped me improve much faster than playing against soccer players whom I was better than. Therefore, the information in this book is so important to guide you as you constantly train with and play against other good players. This will force you to grow into a much better soccer player. If you are reading this book, then you clearly care about getting better at soccer and want to figure out how to train with and play against the best of the best. Using the knowledge in this book will ensure you make the team easily.

Before the Tryout

Chapter 1

Nervous vs. Excited

The famous TEDx speaker and author, Simon Sinek, made a terrific observation when he was watching the 2012 London Olympics. After each athlete's performance, they were asked the same question by interviewers: "Were you nervous?" Each of the athletes had the same response: "No, I was excited."

This is likely because the signs of nervousness and excitement are exactly the same—your heart starts racing, your hands get clammy, and you start visualizing the future. *"The best of the best athletes learned to interpret what their body was telling them not as nerves, but as excitement,"* **says Simon Sinek.** Therefore, use this to your advantage if you want to improve your mindset dramatically for the tryout and even after you have already made the team by reframing your body's feelings. This change in wording has had a huge impact on me for the better and I want to reveal this secret to help you.

Your body physically reacts to nervousness and excitement in the same way. They both create an adrenaline rush. So, why not use the word that increases your performance, instead of the one that decreases it? Punch fear in the face by calling your nerves "excitement!" Instead of saying, "I am nervous to try out for a good team," say, "I am excited to try out for a good team." When using positive self-talk, make sure you always state why you are excited. This will frame your pre-tryout or pre-game jitters in a way that will help your mind be calm and at ease as you try to make the team.

Therefore, change your narrative to make sure you are at ease mentally when trying out. The adrenaline rush you experience is your body's way of getting you ready for the tryout and game time. Understand its importance but avoid focusing on it. Once the tryout starts, that feeling will go away after a few minutes, and you will easily become focused on what you must do in the game. Then, you will no longer think about how you feel and will be able to play to the best of your abilities. Remember, instead of nerves, fear, and stress, view your body's feelings as "excitement." If you want to be an Olympic-level athlete, then mimic and mirror the athletes that are already there. If Olympic athletes are saying they are "excited," then so should you!

Chapter 2

How to Prepare for the Tryout

To make it easier for the coaches to select you for their team, you must start preparing for the tryout as early as you can. **Starting your training two days before the tryout will help you very little and may even leave you sore and unable to perform at your best, whereas starting your training two months before the tryout will give you more time to succeed.** Obviously, months of training will go a long way to ensure you make the team, but assuming that your tryout is fast approaching, and you are reading this book a week or two before your tryout, then you should only focus on the most important things necessary to make the team.

To know what to focus on in the last few days before the tryout, make sure you find out the structure of the tryout. Ask people who have tried out for the team in previous years, or, if you can talk to the coach directly, then ask them what the tryout will look like. Once you know what you will need to work on, you can practice these skills in the weeks or months leading up to the tryout. By practicing the exact things you will be tested on, you can improve your abilities by 10-20%. This can make the difference between an okay performer and a stand-out performer.

For example, in my high school tryout, we had a timed sprint, a two-mile run, a dribbling drill, and plenty of 1v1s. Therefore, every other day leading up to the tryout, I would train and focus on these exact things. This helped me make the junior varsity team in my sophomore year—even though there were several other players who were definitely better at soccer than me and did not get selected for the team. However, it was not very obvious to the coach that they were better because I took the time to build my skills in the specific drills we needed to perform at the tryout. I looked just as good—and sometimes better—than many other players who were better overall but were lazy in their preparations for the tryout.

When they were going through the dribbling drill, it was their first time. On the other hand, it was probably my 50th time going through the drill, but the coaches did not know that. To the coaches, it was my first time, too, because it was the first one they saw me perform.

I used this same mindset when preparing for the varsity tryout at the beginning of my senior year. I came in first place on the one-mile run against 50 or so other players in my group because I trained for the one-mile run three times per week for the entire summer.

However, it is important that your training does not prevent you from performing at your best during the tryout. I made this mistake before my junior year tryout for the varsity team. Several days before the tryout, I performed an intense leg work out of 15 sets of squats. The next morning, I woke up and was not feeling very sore because the delayed-onset muscle soreness (DOMS) had not yet set in. I spent that day doing soccer drills for several hours, and, by the end of the day, I could not walk anymore. Literally! My knees kept buckling as I attempted to walk.

Sadly, for the next week or so, I could not walk correctly. This happened because I did not time my preparation well enough during my efforts to become more fit and ensure I had a good tryout. The first day that I could finally walk again was the first day of the tryout. I had to run a two-mile. Needless to say, it did not go so well. However, despite my poor performance in the two-mile, I still made the team because I was well-prepared for the other drills in the tryout.

Therefore, take at least a day or two before the tryout to let your body recover fully and minimize the chance of any injuries right before the tryout. If you absolutely must do something, then focus on active recovery, like stretching, foam rolling, massages, mobility movements, and/or mild yoga, which are all concepts discussed in the *Understand Soccer* series book, *Soccer Fitness*.

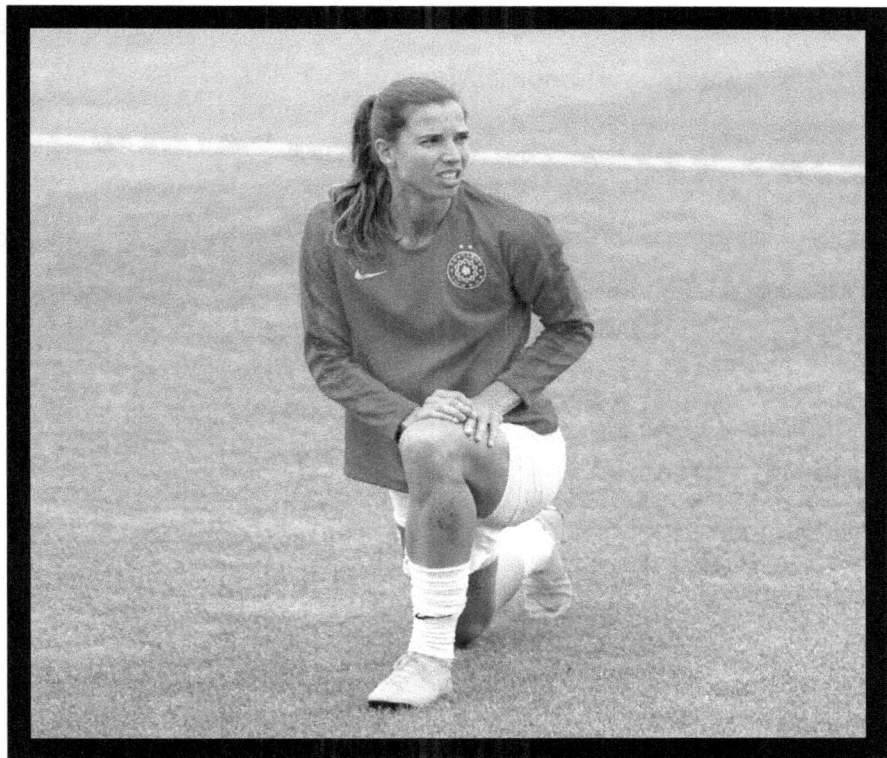

In summary, make your tryout winnable! Even a week or two of prior preparation will make you stand out from the crowd significantly more than if you did not prepare at all.

Consider these key things to put your best foot forward:

1) Understand the format of the tryout so that you can prepare for it appropriately.

2) Practice the drills that you will be tested on.

3) Avoid weight-training the week before the tryout, especially your legs.

4) Take a day or two off before the tryout. Only focus on active recovery if you must do something.

YouTube: If you would like to see a video on how to prepare for your tryouts, then consider watching the *Understand Soccer* YouTube video: *How to Prepare for a Soccer Tryout*.

Chapter 3

Get a Good Night's Sleep

You have a tryout tomorrow, and you cannot fall asleep. You are lying there, thinking about the next day, and seemingly, hours go by without you getting any rest. So, how do you turn your brain off to make sure you are well-rested?

To start, you can try the military method of sleeping. In Sharon Ackerman's popular book, *Relax and Win: Championship Performance*, she describes the U.S. Navy Pre-Flight School's routine to help pilots fall asleep in under two minutes. Pilots often have odd working hours each day and need to fall asleep quickly whenever they have the time to sleep. The pilots trained using the military method for a few weeks before realizing its full effects, but after that, they could even fall asleep after drinking caffeinated beverages and while hearing gunfire in the background!

Step by Step: The Military Sleeping Method

1) Relax your face, including your tongue.
2) Drop your shoulders to release the tension and let your hands drop to the side of your body while lying on your back.
3) Exhale from your chest.

4) Relax your legs, thighs, and calves.

5) Clear your mind for 10 seconds by imagining nothing.

6) Then, try mentally saying the words "don't think" over and over.

7) Within a minute, you should fall asleep!

Personally, I use a more streamlined method in which I focus on turning off my mind. As a child and a young adult, I found it very difficult to fall asleep, as I suffered from a constantly racing mind that was always worrying about the next day's events. However, since figuring out how to turn off my mind, I average about 360 great nights of restful sleep per year. This has given me a large advantage over my competitors because I rarely go through the day feeling exhausted and tired. Remember, I am not a sleep doctor. I am simply a person that went from being someone who had a tough time falling asleep most nights to being someone who is a better sleeper than anyone else I know by a large margin.

My method to turn off my mind is simply looking up with my eyes shut. Yes, it is that simple! By focusing on looking up, you can clear other thoughts from your mind. Also, because you are doing this while your eyes are shut, you will not have any distractions in your room that may affect your sleep. This may sound too easy to you but do not knock it until you try it a few times! I can now fall asleep quickly nearly every night, a few minutes after my head hits the pillow. Additionally, I can even fall asleep quickly when spending nights out of my usual bedroom, such as in a hotel room. After all, it is not fun when you lay down to fall asleep with 8 hours to sleep and end up only obtaining 6.5 hours of sleep.

Age	Optimal Average # of Hours of Sleep
0-8	9-11 Hours
9-12	8-10 Hours
13-17	8-9 Hours
18-65	7-9 Hours
65+	8-9 Hours

The next step is to aim for eight hours of sleep the night before your tryout. Therefore, you should aim to go to bed about eight-and-a-half hours before you need to wake up to ensure you have plenty of time to fall asleep. Avoid eating too much before bed, as this will inhibit deep sleep, and definitely avoid drinking a lot of water! Having to wake up during the middle of the night to use the restroom will increase the chance that you will not fall back to sleep and therefore will not have a restful night's sleep.

Additionally, avoid doing activities that will prevent you from slowing your mind enough to drift off shortly after your head hits the pillow.

Some of these activities to avoid include:

1) Working out.

2) Being on your phone or computer.

3) Consuming caffeine right before bedtime.

4) Getting into an argument.

5) Watching a horror movie.

If you want an entire guide on how to become an amazing sleeper, wake up feeling well-rested every day, and ensure that you become a success in soccer (and in the rest of your life), then grab a copy of the *Understand Soccer* series book, *Soccer Sleep*. This book alone can help give you amazing sleep every night that will make the rest of your life a whole lot easier!

Chapter 4

What to Eat Before and After the Tryout

Your nutrition leading up to and after the tryout can have a significant impact on how well you perform. The trick to ensure your nutrition is top-notch is to plan it. If you fail to plan, then you plan to fail! Let us discuss what and when you should eat leading up to and after your tryout is completed.

What to Eat the Night Before Your Tryout

Before bedtime, you should have a slower-digesting meal, so be sure to consume foods that are high in fiber, fat, and protein. Some examples of these are nuts, seeds, meat, and different kinds of nut butters (e.g., almond butter, cashew butter, and, to a lesser extent, peanut butter). Also, vegetables are always great to eat! Personally, I eat five servings of vegetables a day because they help keep me full longer. Vegetables also contain vitamins, minerals, antioxidants, and phytonutrients that help you recover quicker, keep you feeling better, and maintain steady blood sugar levels, so your energy levels do not spike and crash.

Additionally, if you are not lactose intolerant, then before bedtime is one of the two best times to consume dairy products.

Cheese, Greek yogurt, whole milk (preferably organic), and cottage cheese will do a terrific job of supplying muscle-repairing nutrients to your body for most of the night. This is because dairy's milk protein is made up of 20% whey protein and 80% casein protein. Casein protein takes up to seven hours to digest, which makes it a great pre-bedtime protein to help your body recover and gain strength while you sleep.

Generally, it is a good recommendation to avoid food with a lot of carbohydrates (i.e., carbs) right before bedtime because the carbohydrates can spike your blood sugar levels. Spiked blood sugar levels can make it more difficult to fall asleep and will increase the chance that the food you just ate will be stored as fat rather than be used as fuel.

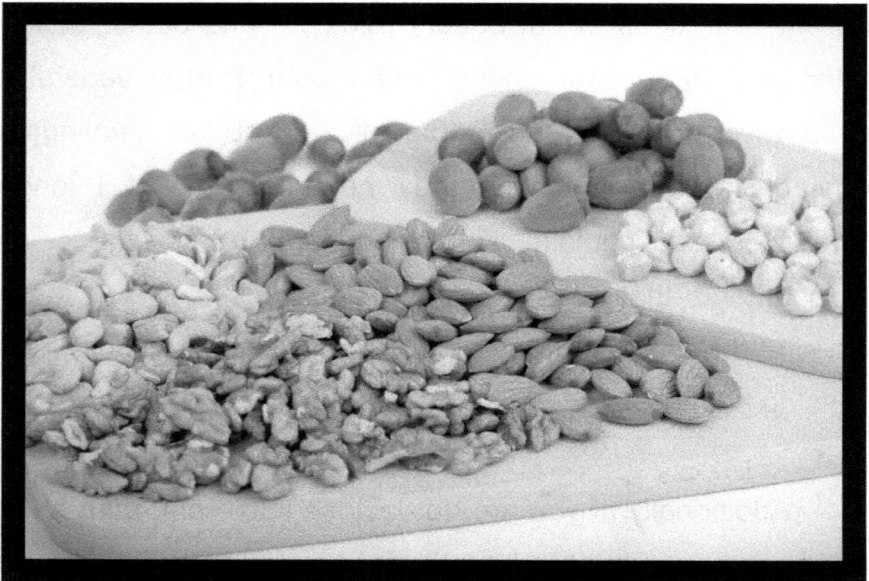

What to Eat the Morning of the Tryout

Upon awakening on the day of your tryout, your body has used up most of its glycogen (i.e., blood sugar) stores throughout the night, so you will need to consume foods that are higher in carbohydrates. Some examples are fruits, vegetables, and healthy grains, such as quinoa, brown rice, sweet potatoes, steel-cut oatmeal, and organic bread. These carbohydrates are very beneficial to replenish your body's blood sugar stores and to give you the energy you need to function appropriately until your next meal.

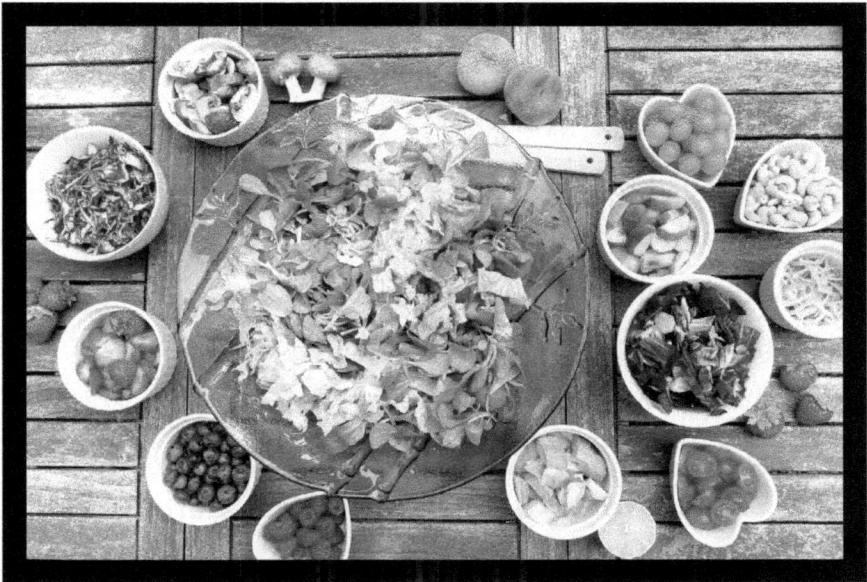

There is a common misconception in the athletic world that you are supposed to "carb up" the night before a game. For example, many teams will have a pasta dinner the night before a game, thinking this will help them get enough carbs to be fully fueled for the game the next day. However, in reality, eating some carbohydrates is a good thing if you just finished a training session, but you do not need to eat three bowls of pasta the night before a game. Eating too many carbs the night before a game will only increase the chance that it will be stored in your body as fat.

Also, a good recommendation for the morning of the tryout is to a consume some protein. However, avoid dairy products! Furthermore, there are better options than nuts, seeds, and beef during the morning of your tryout. Instead, eat some eggs or faster digesting sources of protein like chicken, turkey, or fish. Personally, scrambled eggs work best for me because I can prepare them with onions (i.e., a vegetable) and make several servings at once. This is great to have as a healthy grab-and-go choice in the morning when you are often hurried and rushed to get out the door.

What to Eat Before Your Tryout Starts

It is beneficial to consume carbs closer to the tryout, but this depends on how well your body digests food, and how empty or full you prefer your stomach to be when playing soccer. Often, 2-4 hours before the start of a tryout is an ideal time to take in more carbohydrates in the form of the following:

1) Faster-digesting vegetables, such as carrots.
2) Fruits, such as apples, bananas, or watermelon.
3) Carbs, such as quinoa, sweet potatoes, or brown rice.

Furthermore, you should consume fish, turkey, or grilled chicken to ensure you have some protein to keep you more full for longer.

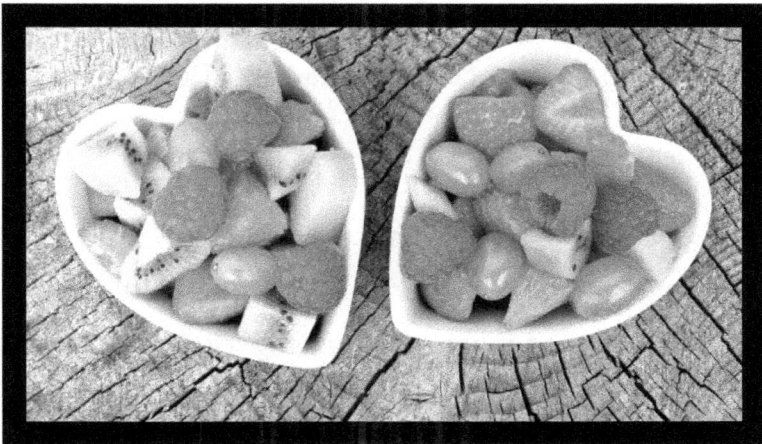

Should You Consume a Pre-Workout Supplement?

The decision to take a pre-workout supplement before a tryout will vary from person to person. Personally, I would take a high-quality pre-workout supplement to give me additional energy during the tryout. After all, it is very important to show off your skills and abilities. If you lack the energy that you need to perform in a tryout, then it will be more difficult to succeed at making the team. In my estimation, a scoop of a pre-workout supplement before the tryout will increase your chance of making the team by 10-15%.

I would not recommend at least 80% of the pre-workout supplements on the market. They are filled with artificial colors, flavors, and sweeteners, which make it seem like you are getting more for your money. In reality, you are getting a bunch of chemicals that will only lead to long-term problems. Instead, go for a pre-workout supplement with only a few high-powered ingredients. One of my recommendations is Pure Pump.

Pure Pump has all the trusted ingredients that a pre-workout supplement should have—without any of the fluff. All three products are for both men and women. *(Note that I am not sponsored by any of these companies; I just really like these products because they do not add unnecessary ingredients.)*

Personally, I consume the unflavored versions of these products, but they do taste a bit metallic, so you may prefer the flavored versions. One scoop works well for children, and two scoops is the recommended serving size for an adult. Make sure to dissolve them into at least eight ounces of water.

However, given that I am not a licensed physician, please consult your doctor first before trying any pre-workout supplements on your own.

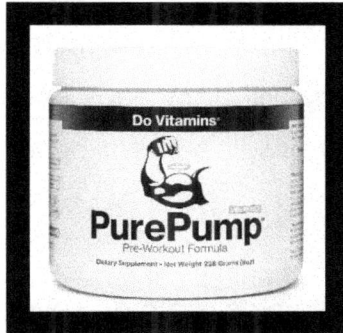

How Much Water Should You Drink?

According to the National Collegiate Athletic Association (NCAA), here is the recommended amount of water to consume:

When:	Ounces:	Ounces-to-Bottles:
2-3 Hours Before the Tryout	16 ounces	About 1 Regular-Sized Bottle
15 Minutes Before the Tryout	8 ounces	About 1/2 Regular-Sized Bottle
During the Tryout	4 ounces every 15-20 minutes	About 2-3 Large Gulps (1/4 of a Regular-Sized Bottle)
After the Tryout	16-20 ounces	1 to 1-1/4 Regular-Sized Bottles or 1 Large Bottle

What to Eat After the Tryout

Anytime you use your muscles, your muscle fibers break down. However, when they are provided with enough quality nutrition and rest, they will grow back even stronger. The next time you use them, you will perform better, quicker, and more efficiently.

Because most tryouts are over several days, it is ideal to take in nutrition after each tryout to help your muscles recover and grow. Foods that are high in carbohydrates and fast-digesting proteins are good to consume after a tryout for optimal muscle recovery. One example of this is organic milk. Although research shows alternating views on lactose, having some organic milk or a whey protein shake with non-GMO dextrose is beneficial after each tryout is completed. You should take in enough carbohydrates to spike your blood sugar after a tryout, game, or workout so that your body will better use the protein that you take in.

Whey protein is recommended because it is one of the most bio-available and quickest digesting proteins. If you drink milk, it has milk protein, which is 20% whey protein and 80% casein protein. It is essential that if you have more physical activities later in the day or a second portion of the tryout that same day, take in enough carbohydrates to replenish your glycogen. It is critical to minimize the amount of fat and fiber that you take in during the post-workout 30-minute window after a tryout because fiber and fat are slower digesting. They slow the absorption of vitamins, minerals, and nutrients. Avoid very dense foods like spinach or peanut butter unless there is absolutely nothing else that you can consume. Something healthy is better than nothing.

Then, consume a meal similar to the meal you ate a few hours before the tryout started. Include a meat, a fruit, a vegetable, and a carb to help your body recover from the intense tryout.

Example Tryout Meal Plan for a 3 p.m. Start Time

Night Before the Tryout:

½ cup of nuts (protein)
4 ounces of organic cheese (protein)
1-2 cups of leafy greens (vegetable)
1 cup of Greek yogurt or cottage cheese (protein)

(Note: The nuts, cheese, and Greek yogurt/cottage cheese also contain some carbohydrates and fats too. These are slow digesting and will aid in nighttime recovery.)

Breakfast (8 AM):

3 eggs (protein)
½ sautéed onion (vegetable)
½ cup of oatmeal (carb)
1 orange (optional additional carb)

Lunch (noon):

8 ounces of grilled chicken breast (protein)
1 cup of carrots (vegetable)
1 apple (fruit – carb)
1-2 slices of organic bread (carb)

Snack (as needed):

1 banana (fruit – carb)
2 organic rice cakes (carb)

Pre-Tryout (30 minutes before the tryout):

1-2 scoops of pre-workout supplement (additional energy)

Post-Tryout (5 PM):

1 scoop of whey protein isolate (muscle recovery and growth)
1-2 cups of milk or water (muscle recovery and growth)
5 grams of creatine (muscle recovery and growth)

Dinner (6 PM):

8 ounces of poultry, beef, chicken, or fish (protein)
1 cup of broccoli (vegetable)
1 cup of blueberries (fruit – carb)
1 sweet potato (carb)

30 Minutes Before Bedtime:

½ cup of nuts (protein)
4 ounces of organic cheese (protein)
1-2 cups of leafy greens (vegetable)
1 cup of Greek yogurt or cottage cheese (protein)

(Note: This is a great meal plan for an adult. If you are a child or are reading this to help your child, then cut the portion sizes roughly in half. Make substitutions where necessary, such as substituting one fruit or vegetable for another. For example, eating watermelon instead of a banana is terrific and so is eating celery instead of onions.)

What if You are Not Used to Eating Healthy?

Remember that if you have not eaten nutritiously for the last several months, then changing your eating habits the day before a tryout will not cure all your ailments—but it is a great place to start! Nutrition compounds, and good nutrition can set you up for success both in soccer and in life. An ancient Chinese proverb states, *"The best time to plant a tree is 20 years ago; the second-best time is now."* The best time to act is in the present. The past is behind us and cannot be undone, but putting something off until the future only increases the chance that it will *never* get done. Therefore, start now! Make a plan or a system that is easy to stick with. This will make it easier for you to make the right food choices consistently and take massive action towards becoming extremely healthy, fit, and confident.

If you want more information on eating well to improve your performances, focusing on the areas of nutrition that will bring you the biggest results in the least amount of time, and how Lionel Messi and Cristiano Ronaldo eat to prepare for a game, then grab the *Understand Soccer* series book, *Soccer Nutrition*.

During the Tryout

Chapter 5

Your First Impression

The sociolinguist Albert Mehrabian conducted comprehensive research on communication in which he found that in a face-to-face encounter, 55% of the message is transmitted through the speaker's appearance and body language, 38% comes from the speaker's vocal tone, pacing, and inflection, and 7% comes from the words used by the speaker. In other words, in the first 7-27 seconds after you meet a coach, **93% of your first impression is *not* determined by the words you say**. Although this seems like a flaw, it is terrific to understand and use to ensure you put your best foot forward while dramatically increasing your chances of making the team.

Though many people wish coaches could see past first impressions and only judge a player on their abilities, this is not how the soccer world works. Coaches are humans just like you and are very quick to stand by their first impressions of who they think are "good" and who they are unlikely to choose for the team, even though coaches believe they are completely fair and unbiased. **Because you now understand this flaw in human nature that people tend to place too much emphasis on deciding whether we like someone when we first meet them, you can use this knowledge to your advantage by** ensuring you make a great first impression that will set you up for success in the entire tryout.

Here are nine great nonverbal ways to make a positive first impression:

1) **Get to the field early.** Arriving at the field early will make a terrific first impression by showing the coach that you value their time and are not a player who will be late to practices or games. The general rule of thumb before games and practices is to plan to arrive 20 minutes early for each hour of driving you need to do. Therefore, if you have a game that is two hours away, then plan to leave at least two hours and 40 minutes before the game starts to give yourself a cushion. However, because the tryout is arguably more important than a game, you should make sure to leave 30 minutes early for each hour of driving you need to do. Therefore, if the tryout is one hour away, then you should leave one hour and 30 minutes before it starts. If the tryout is only 30 minutes away, then leave at least 45 minutes before it starts. Use the GPS app on your cell phone to avoid any accidents, detours, traffic, or roadwork that could make you late. The coach will not care why you were late, so make sure you show up early to make a good first impression! Arriving at the field early to meet the coach will ensure that you have a better chance of talking with them and making your first impression in a one-on-one conversation before the other players.

Additionally, meeting the coach will make it easier to be calmer when the physically demanding portion of the tryout occurs.

2) **Dress well.** Wear vibrant colors, like highlighter orange, bright yellow, baby blue, etc. If your tryout will be held over multiple days, then aim to keep the same look every day, so you will stand out to the coach and be easier to remember. Sadly, I never even thought about this tip when I was in middle school, high school, and college! It was recently suggested to me by my sister, who made the varsity team at one of the largest high schools in the state as a freshman. Although I never used it, she swears by it, and using it will ensure that you have as many advantages as possible over the other players.

3) **Smile!** A smile is an invitation to talk to you. Given that coaches will need to get to know each player better, smiling will make it easier for you to build a connection with them and communicate that you are friendly and approachable without using any words. The field of Psychology has revealed that when you smile at someone, it will make that person more likely to trust you. Don't you think a coach will want a trustworthy player on their team?

4) **Stand up straight!** Status, power, and even skills on the soccer field are nonverbally conveyed by stature and space. Standing tall, pulling your shoulders back, and holding your

head straight are all signs of confidence, self-esteem, and competence, in soccer and in life.

5) **Always make eye contact.** Looking into a coach's eyes will tell them that you are a confident player who is interested in joining the team. A great way to work on your eye contact is to notice the eye color of every coach on the team.

6) **Raise your eyebrows.** Open your eyes and raise your eyebrows slightly more than normal. This is the universal signal of recognition and acknowledgement. Also, this shows you are excited to meet the coach and coaches prefer picking players who like them.

7) **Shake their hand.** This is the quickest way to establish a good relationship with the coach and one of the most effective. Make sure you have a firm handshake to show the coach you are strong.

8) **Have a great attitude.** Before you meet the coach, make the choice about having the attitude of a player that you think they would want to have on their team. Be energetic to stand out from the other players.

9) **Pay attention!** When the coach calls the players in at the beginning of the first tryout, sprint to them and stand directly in

front of the coach. This is an easy trick to show the coach you are committed to excellence. You will stand out and be much more memorable than the other players who walked or jogged to the circle. Do not hide in the middle of a huddle or go to the back of the group to take a knee. The more times the coach sees you, the better! Additionally, coaches like to be listened to, so if they give you advice, take it and implement it immediately. They want players on their team who will listen.

Look at the following image and see if you can figure out which players are hurting their chances of making a great impression:

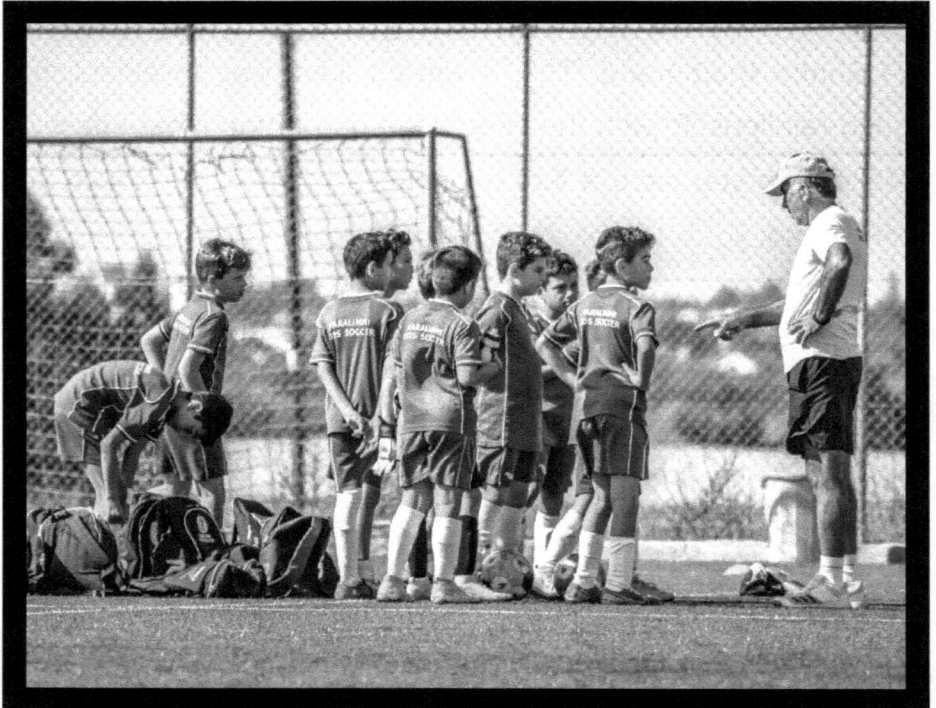

Here is a quick list of common mistakes soccer players make during a tryout:

1) **Slouching.** This expresses a lack of desire to be at the tryout. It is good to lean in to show interest but slouching shows disinterest when the coach is talking. Coaches do not want players who do not want to listen.

2) **Forgetting to Make Eye Contact.** Sometimes, it is difficult to be confident around an adult who may be much older than you. Making and keeping eye contact can seem a bit overwhelming, but if you do not look them in the eyes, it will make you seem very disengaged. If you are shy and cannot bring yourself to look the coach directly in the eyes, then look at the spot on their face directly *between* both eyes. This will make it a lot easier to look at them without having to look them squarely in the eyes; however, to them, it will still seem like you are looking them in the eyes.

3) **Crossing Your Arms.** Whether they are crossed in front of your body, held behind your body, or resting tightly by your sides, if you close your arms, then you are sending the message, "I am unapproachable, I am nervous, I am awkward, and you should not talk to me." Make sure to loosen up your arms, bend them at the elbows, and relax. If you use your hands

while talking, then great! Just avoid being too rigid, which will lead to a poor first impression.

4) **Appearing Lazy.** Remember that the coach will only see your skills a few times over the course of the tryout. Appearing energetic will ensure that you get additional looks, whereas acting lazy, "too cool," or indifferent will make it easier for the coach to reject you because they will think that if you are not taking the tryout seriously, then you probably will not take practices seriously, either.

5) **Being Rude or Mean to Other Players.** Coaches try to create the best atmosphere for their team to make it easier for each of the individual players to grow. Therefore, by belittling others or pointing out others' mistakes, the coach will assume you are a negative person. Coaches already have enough negativity after losses and from parents of the players trying out or who are already on the team. Coaches do not want to add a rude player to their team whose mindset of negativity may affect other players on the team, too.

Remember that making a great first impression is something you can do regardless of whether or not you are good at soccer. There are many things you can do that involve no skill or talent and take very little effort to do. Take advantage of as many of them as you can to make it nearly impossible for the coach to reject you. Remember that having quality soccer skills is important, but when two soccer players have similar skills, a coach will always select the player who does the things mentioned in this chapter.

US Youth Soccer interviewed Ronnie Woodard, the former women's coach of Vanderbilt University. While providing insight on some of the most important tryout questions, she said, *"Coaches are looking for players who make an impact and get their attention. It is very important for players to get the coaches to notice them, and it isn't always easy."* Give yourself an advantage by using the information in this chapter to make sure you get noticed for all the right reasons and make a great first impression.

YouTube: If you would like to see a video on how to make a great first impression, then consider watching the *Understand Soccer* YouTube video: *How to Stand Out at a Soccer Tryout*.

Chapter 6

Be Coachable

As an athlete, you want to make sure you are really approachable and very coachable. Act enthusiastically and show you are having fun. Positivity is magnetic, and coaches want positive and optimistic players on their team. Having the ability to be coached ensures that you will absorb the knowledge that your coaches give you.

We like to think that we know everything, but being open to other people's opinions, ideas, and words of wisdom will make it so that we are even more knowledgeable. **In sports and in life, it is critical to have a growth mindset, in which you are continually seeking new information**, as well as learning new skills, tips, and tricks in all the significant endeavors in your life. Not only is this important on the field but in the classroom and at home, too.

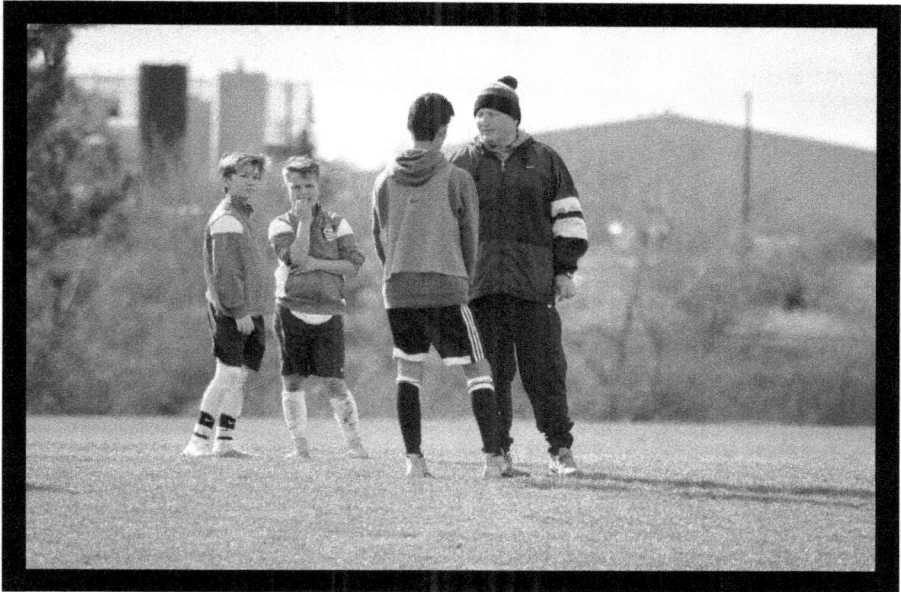

Therefore, anytime the coach gives a piece of information to the entire group, or you specifically, **thank them for the feedback—even if they are giving it in a mean way**. If you want the coach to know that you are coachable because you care about being a better player and making the team, then take action on what they say immediately. This mindset of immediate action will be very obvious to coaches and will show them you are open to their feedback. **Also, remember that it is just feedback, not a personal attack against you.** It is not that they hate you, are trying to tear you down, or want to make you less of a player; instead, it is that they care about you and want you to improve rapidly. If you show that you care about their opinions and immediately implement their teachings, then they will like you even more. As a result, they will select you for their soccer team.

Being coachable means that you are open to coaching—not only from coaches but from other players, too. During the tryout, if another player mentions a good point to you, then say, "Thank you for the feedback." This statement turns what could be an awkward situation into a situation in which you appreciate the other person for helping you become better. Additionally, by having the "last word," you will not lose social status with the other players who are watching the interaction.

However, if a teammate says something very obvious and potentially sarcastic like "take a better touch" or "have better control." Instead of being snide and having a rude comment the coach will probably hear, just say in a non-sarcastic tone, "thank you for the feedback." This shows your emotionally mature enough to take feedback from teammates which reveals to the coach you will be mature enough to take feedback from them. **The phrase "thank you for the feedback" applies in nearly every situation and is easy to remember.**

Next, when others do well in the tryout, congratulate them for a job well done. This shows the coaching staff that you have so much confidence in your own abilities that you are confident enough to congratulate others. Additionally, it shows that you care about the team's success and not just your own. Also, by associating yourself with the other good players, the coach will mentally group you in with the good players which improves your chances of making the team!

Some of this chapter has been excerpted from the first *Understand Soccer* series book, *Soccer Training*. *Soccer Training* is a high-level guide that discusses one important topic in each area of soccer that a soccer player must understand. Therefore, this is a must-read book in the series to make sure you have a well-rounded knowledge in many important things related to your game.

In summary, make sure you show the coach that you are coachable by doing the following:

1) Having a positive attitude.
2) Being open to feedback from the coach and implementing it.
3) Not getting too worried about receiving feedback; instead, just learning from it.
4) Congratulating others for a job well done.

Chapter 7

Communicate!

This is the most important chapter in this book. This one tip alone is worth 10X the price of the book. This tip is a "cheat code" that is the easiest thing to do during a tryout, but it is also the easiest thing to forget. It takes no skill as a soccer player but ensures that you get noticed by the coaches. **The tip is to never stop communicating.**

So, what exactly does it mean to communicate? Well, let us dive into how to communicate effectively during a tryout. **Communicating is best used in any scrimmages, whether those be full-field scrimmages or small-sided games.** Make sure you are constantly directing other people what to do, not in a bossy tone, but in a helpful tone.

Things to say include:

1) "Turn!"
2) "Pressure!"
3) "Take your space!"
4) "Cross the ball!"
5) "Play it backwards!"
6) "Pass it wide!"

7) "Dribble them!"

8) "Lay off the ball!"

9) "Push up the field!"

10) "Man/Woman on!"

11) "Here!"

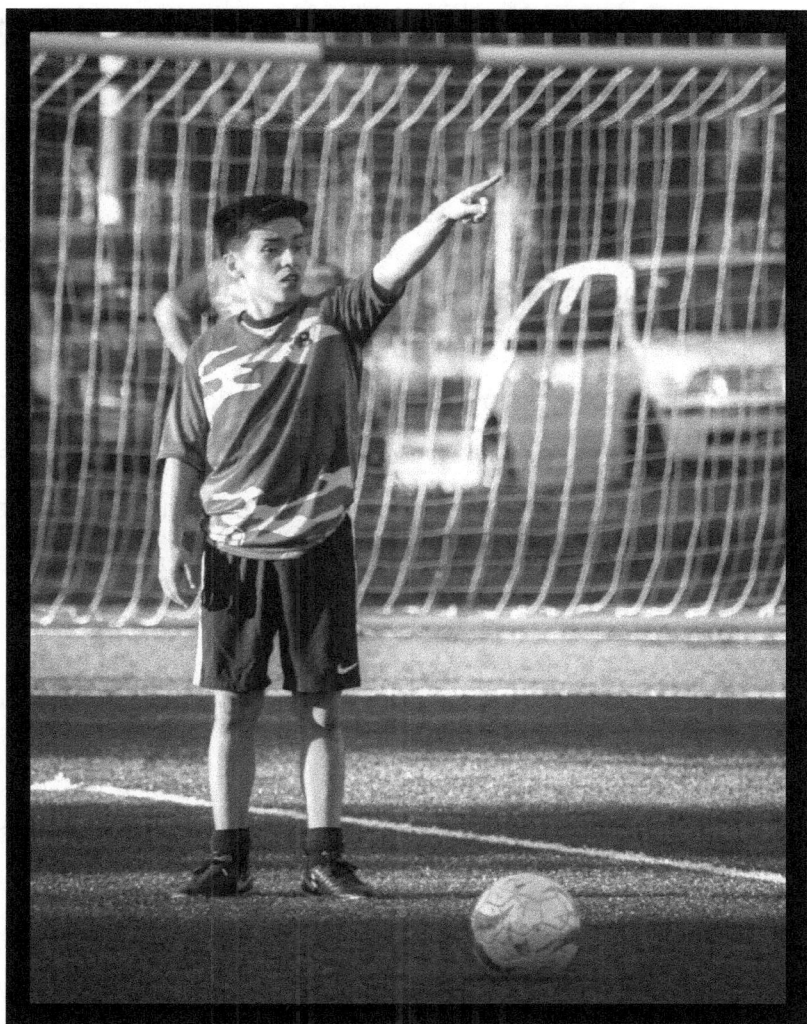

Communicating these things will:

1) Help you and your teammates win the scrimmages in the tryout.

2) Help you get noticed by the coaches because you will stand out as one of the few "talkers."

3) Boost your confidence in other areas of soccer because other players will see you as a leader.

Remember, talking is just as easy to do as it is *not* to do. You need zero foot skills, shooting abilities, or defensive tactics to communicate to others what they should be doing. Remember that because the coach will hear you more, they will also see and notice you more. This does two important things. First, it ensures you get a fair look. Second, it makes it seem like you are working harder and doing more than everyone else because the coach keeps hearing you. The coach associates the players that stand out with being good players, so the easiest way to stand out—even if you are not that good at soccer—is to communicate nonstop.

When I first started posting memes, fun facts, and tips on my **Instagram account, @UnderstandSoccer**, I revealed this one tip to Wes, the first person who asked me for advice on how to succeed in his tryout. Keep in mind that I only messaged Wes through the app and sent him a quick one-minute video clip explaining the concept. That was it—a one-minute clip! He took the advice, implemented it, and made the team. He then told me the good news.

I said to him, "It was all your hard work that got you to this point."

He responded, "Although that definitely gave me some abilities to hold my own at the tryout, your one tip was the reason I got on the team."

I countered, "No, it was not; there are so many other factors; certainly, it was you."

He kindly replied, "The tip that you said would be the most important—about communicating a ton—was the exact reason the coach decided to choose me for the team. Thanks for all your help!"

It blew me away how effective this one tip can be for a soccer player worried about making the team. It was great to see this tip work for the first person whom I revealed it to.

I knew this tip on communicating worked perfectly for me. Using it, I was able to get noticed by a coaching staff that selected me, a soccer player at the time that had never played club soccer before. They selected me over 50 or so other soccer players, most of which had played club soccer for years. This chapter on directing your teammates by communicating is that powerful.

Therefore, make sure you communicate as loudly as you can. Remember that not only do you need the players whom you are directing to hear you, but **you also really need the coach to hear you. Often, coaches are talking with other coaches or players on the sideline, so they are not looking at you. By communicating very loudly, they do not have to see you to know that you are working hard on the field.** Again, the more instances in which they notice you are doing something good—like communicating—the more they will associate you with the "good players" and select you for the team.

YouTube: If you would like to see a video on how to make a great first impression, then consider watching the *Understand Soccer* YouTube video: *Tricks to Stand Out at Tryouts*.

Chapter 8

Try Out for the Position You Want to Play

Typically, a large percentage of the tryout will be spent scrimmaging. No matter whether these are small-sided or full-field scrimmages, you should expect that you will have to play and perform in them. Therefore, make sure you are adamant, persistent, and decisive about playing the position you want to play in a scrimmage! In this chapter, we will discuss how to communicate where you want to play effectively, when to remain persistent, and when *not* to demand that you play your preferred position.

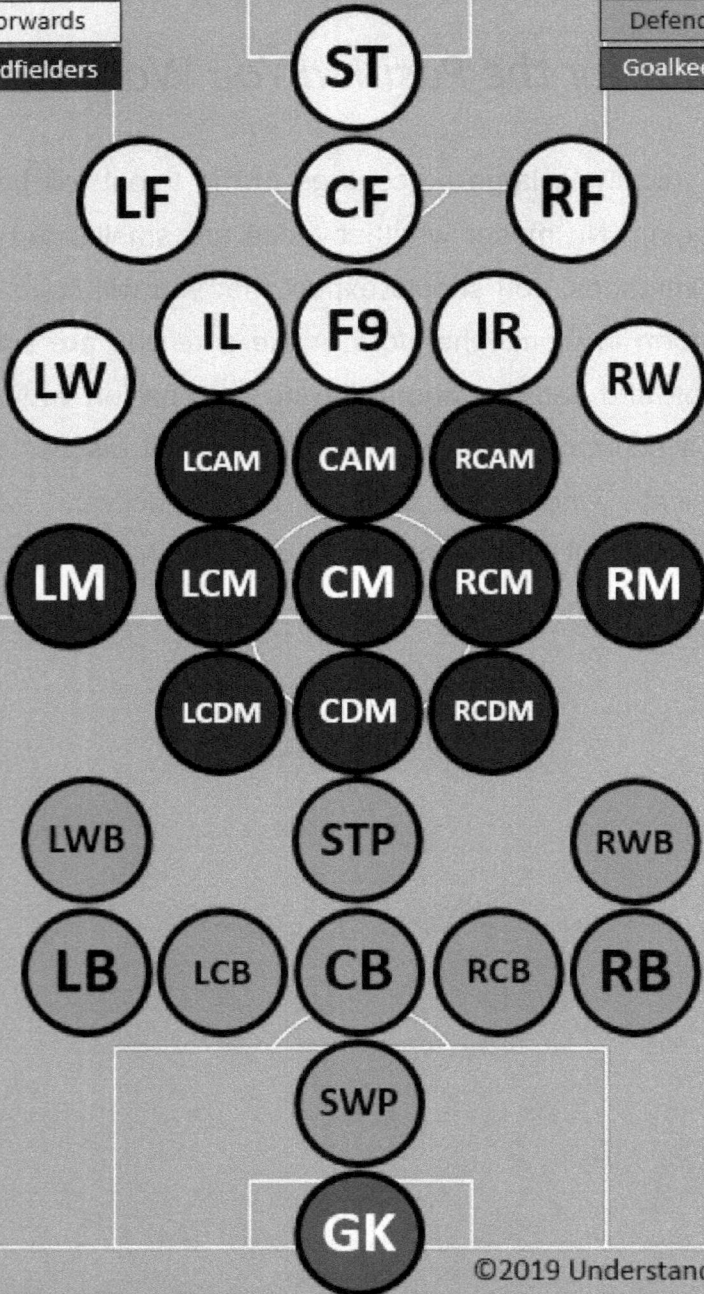

Forwards
Midfielders
Defenders
Goalkeeper

ST
LF CF RF
IL F9 IR
LW RW
LCAM CAM RCAM
LM LCM CM RCM RM
LCDM CDM RCDM
LWB STP RWB
LB LCB CB RCB RB
SWP
GK

©2019 Understand, LLC

First, the coach will often discuss the previous drill and then will say, "We are going to scrimmage." If the coach asks each player what position they want to play, then this is the perfect time to tell them your preferred position. If the coach asks you if you will play anywhere else, then you must weigh your options. **Specifically, if this is a tryout for a club team, and there are plenty of other club teams to try out for, then you can be much more forceful in saying that you only want to play your favored position. However, if this is a tryout for something like a high school team, and you'll either make it and be on the team or will not make it and cannot play soccer for the next several months, then making the team may be more important to you than playing your preferred position.** Here, you can let the coach know your preferred position and add the statement, "I am also willing to play in another position if it would best help the team." Again, this must be a decision that you make before the tryout. Ask yourself, "What is more important to me: playing my preferred position or making the team?"

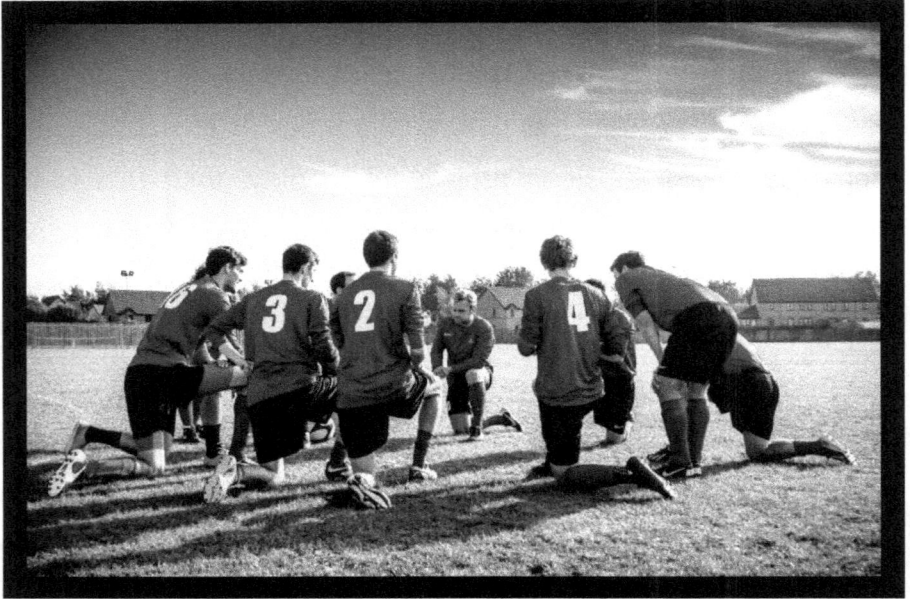

However, in many instances, the coach will not assign positions as a tactic to see where each of the players will start by letting them pick their own spots. Often, shy players will start on the bench. You do not want to start on the bench because the coach will most likely associate you with the bench players. The coach will associate each player with the position they initially line up in. Also, many players who are not persistent about playing their desired position will end up as an outside midfielder or outside defender. This is a good thing if you prefer one of those spots. **However, if you want to be more centrally located in the defensive, midfield, or attacking portions of the field, then as soon as the coach finishes talking about the scrimmage, you need to make sure to loudly say "I'll play forward," or "I will be a center midfielder," or "I've got**

center back." By saying the position you want out loud, you will have "dibs" on the position. This is important because it will be a lot harder for someone else to take that spot from you if you have already verbally claimed it in front of everyone.

Though it may seem a bit awkward and unnecessary to call out the position you want as teams are getting decided, it is even more awkward for you, a forward, getting stuck as a defender and getting beat constantly because that is not where you have developed skills or a lot of experience. This would likely lead to the coach having a bad impression of you because you were not forceful enough to be in your preferred position. **Therefore, loudly calling out your preferred position and being persistent about playing it is not nearly as scary as having a bad tryout in the wrong position and not making the team.**

Therefore, it is important to be very persistent if another player asks to play in the spot you have already claimed. Make sure you use the tryout as a platform to show off your abilities. The major reason you are at the tryout is to help yourself make the team, not to be walked all over by someone else who is also trying to make the team and wants to play in the same position as you. **Do not worry if you offend someone else by saying "no, I am going to start here," if they ask to start in the spot you have already claimed.**

On the other hand, if a member of the coaching staff asks you to switch spots, then you must weigh your options again. If you are trying out for several teams and only want to play in a forward role, then inform the coach of this by saying, "I care a lot about helping this team, and I can do that best in this position." Do not come across as disrespectful or rude, but make sure the coach knows you must play in this spot. Often, a coach will be impressed that you can communicate what you want and handle yourself with class.

However, if you really want to make the team—even more than you want to play in your preferred role—then say, "I would be glad to play that position for the time being, and my preferred position is (your ideal position)." Use the word "and" not "but" because saying "but" will come across as a complaint, and coaches rarely want complainers on their team. Saying "and" merely reveals that you are stating a fact that you want the coach to know.

Then, move to the position that the coaching staff has asked of you. If you end up in that position for a while, just remind the coach, "I've been playing in that position for a while. Could you put me in as a (your ideal position)? I can contribute more to the team in that position." If you say this politely, then coaches often will move you to your ideal position. **However,**

how long you stay in your preferred position depends on how well you play there.

In summary, make sure you:

1) Weigh which is more important: playing on the team or playing in the position you prefer.
2) Loudly call "dibs" on the position you want after the coach is finished talking about the scrimmage.
3) Do not back down to another player who is looking to take the spot that you have claimed.

If you are unsure what position would be the best fit for you, then grab a copy of the *Understand Soccer* series book, *Soccer Positions*, to learn what skills are needed in the 30+ possible positions on the field.

Chapter 9

Show Off Your Strengths

Do not think of tryouts as practice. In practice, you should be slightly outside your comfort zone to learn and grow, while occasionally making mistakes that you can then use as stepping stones to become more successful. This mindset is not appropriate for a tryout because you generally should not look to gain better skills and abilities during a tryout. Instead, you should focus only on showcasing what you are best at to ensure that the coach will see you in a positive light and will be more likely to select you for the team.

Therefore, for a tryout, you must:

1) Determine your strengths.
2) Showcase your strengths.
3) Hide your weaknesses.

First, start by determining what your strengths are. This is best done at least a couple weeks before your tryout takes place. Specifically, giving yourself enough time for a few more individual practices before the tryout can ensure that you work on exactly what you aim to show off in the tryout. **To determine your strengths, think about which parts of soccer are most**

fun for you, and the areas you are often complimented on. Here is where you will easily find your strengths.

For example, you may enjoy defending in 1v1s and often get compliments from coaches, parents, and teammates on your ability to pass. In this case, you should make sure you are playing in a defensive or center defensive midfield role to ensure you can show your strengths, and the coach will labels you as a "good defender" or a "good passer." Maybe you are great at beating defenders in 1v1s and have a powerful shot. In this case, you should look to practice your strengths leading up to the tryout, so you will be comfortable in an attacking center midfield or forward role, and the coach will label you as a "goal-scorer."

Think of at least two strengths that you want to highlight in the tryout, so the coach who is making the selections for the team will see you in the best light. **Determining your strengths a few weeks before your tryout will give you enough time to practice your preferred skills.**

Finally, avoid situations that reveal your weaknesses. This is not to say that having areas that need improvement is a bad thing, nor is it to say that you should avoid developing any of your weaknesses. However, a tryout is not the place to try new skills or attempt things outside your comfort zone unless absolutely required. The time for that is in practice, after you have already made the team. Coaches only have limited time to make a decision about each player, and they rarely change their mind after they have decided if you are good enough for the team. By trying new things and wanting to appear flashy, you will increase your chance of messing up, and the coach may automatically label you as someone who makes "poor decisions," and thus you will likely not make the team. This label is hard to change once the coach has made up their mind, so be sure to avoid it. **The trick is to not show off, just to showcase your strengths. Therefore, think of at least two things you are not good at doing and avoid those in the tryout.**

For example, a defender may have weak foot skills and a bad shot. In this case, the defender should hide those inabilities by playing strong defense and passing the ball to a teammate as soon as they get it. If you lack speed, then avoid getting in foot races with other players. Instead, use your foot skills, take open shots, and pass the ball whenever you cannot outpace the defender. Again, it cannot be emphasized enough that working on your weaknesses until they do not hold you back is very important in your soccer career. However, you must avoid displaying your weaknesses in a tryout. This is not the time to "take one for the team" by putting yourself in poor situations while making it easier for others to shine. That kind of behavior is admirable, but it will not help you make the team.

In summary, your strengths are what will get you on the team. Ideally, a few weeks before the tryout, you should determine your strengths, which will give you enough time to work on them. Your focus in the tryout should be to impress the coach, and the easiest way to achieve this and get a spot on the team is to make sure that they see your well-developed skills. Therefore, only seek situations in a tryout that will highlight your skills and abilities and save the development of your weaknesses for practice after you have already made the team.

Chapter 10

The Big 3 Foot Skills: Jab Steps, Self-Passes, and Shot Fakes

Bruce Lee, the famous martial artist and philosopher, once said, "*I fear not the man who has practiced 10,000 kicks once, but I fear the man who has practiced one kick 10,000 times.*" What he is saying is do not settle with just dabbling in many skills across many different areas; instead, you should strive to be the best in only one thing. **In soccer, this means that you must pick one skill for each of the different circumstances in a game that you may encounter and develop those skills—and only those!**

Please keep in mind that this chapter is especially geared towards midfielders and forwards. If you are a defender, avoid using foot skills in nearly all situations at a tryout because coaches rarely like defenders who dribble the ball too much. The Big 3 foot skills that are recommended for soccer players to develop are the jab step, self-pass, and shot fake. If you subscribed to the UnderstandSoccer.com email list, then this chapter will look familiar. If not, it is highly recommended to subscribe to it for tips, tricks, tweaks, and techniques emailed to you about one time per week after the first week of emails.

First, the jab step goes by many names: the shoulder drop, the fake, the fake-and-take, the feint, the body feint, or whatever else you would like to call it. The name is not essential but mastering the skill is crucial. This skill is by far the best attacking move to use when a defender is backpedaling, and you are looking to dribble past them. Now, keep in mind that any skill in this situation should be used to throw the defender off-balance for a split-second, during which the defender will think you are going in one direction, when you really intend to take the ball in another direction. However, the explosive change of speed after the skill has been performed will buy you more time than performing the jab step with the appropriate form. **A good jab step is performed with the ball starting outside your shoulder, then turning your toe down and in to make it look like you will push the ball.**

Some soccer players may prefer to use the scissor or the step over in this game situation. **Yet, the jab step allows you to make no contact whatsoever with the ball and does not require any extra body positioning that involves additional steps similar to that of a scissor.** Additionally, this is not the correct time to do a step over. A correctly performed scissor requires you to step your plant foot past the ball, so you can turn at the hips, which will allow the ball to roll through your legs while the defender is off-balance, thereby allowing you to push the ball and attack in the opposite direction. In a scissor, the extra step required to position your body past the ball correctly will take extra time versus a jab step.

Let us use a very well-known player to demonstrate this further - Lionel Messi. Some would argue that he is or is not the best soccer player ever, however, there is not much of an argument when someone says he is the best dribbler in the world. **When you watch him, it does not look like he is doing a bunch of skills to dribble past the defenders since it looks so effortless. However, upon further inspection, you will see that he is using the most efficient skills, which he has perfected.** He uses the most efficient skills to score more goals, tally more assists, and increase the chance that his team wins.

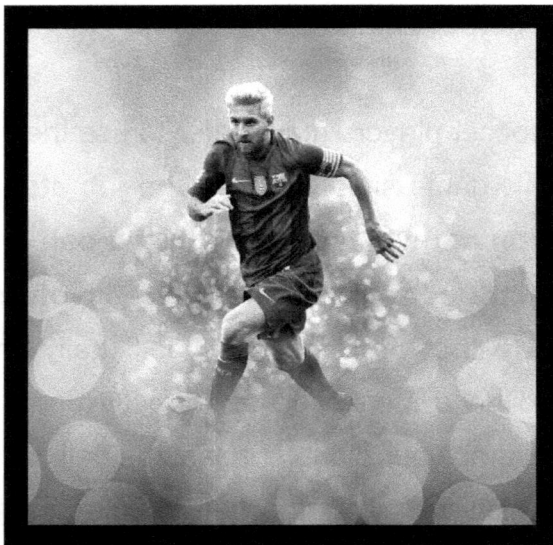

Again, this is not to say that the other skills are bad; it is just that they are not as likely to work. Think about it this way: If you do a jab step, you will have a 90% success rate, whereas when you perform a scissor, you will have an 80% success rate. **Therefore, the jab step is a better option because it takes less time and you will have a higher percentage of success.**

Let me give you a personal example. As a trainer at one of the Next Level Training soccer summer camps, a player named Emily followed my advice in a drill that we were doing. The drill was simply 1v1s, and she had to travel to the other side of the grid for a point. Emily did the same jab step nine times in a row, and it worked every single time.

Next, the self-pass is a very effective skill when the defender is reaching in for the ball. Anytime they are reaching towards you to take the ball away; it naturally means their momentum is going towards you, and your momentum is going in the opposite direction. This means you do not need to fake the ball one way and take it another way when the opposing player is lunging toward the ball. Simply move the ball out of the way. The self-pass is also known as an "L," an "Iniesta," or a "La Croqueta." It is as easy as passing the ball from one foot to the other straight across the defender's body—**not across your own body**. Going across the defender's body is critical because the ball should not travel diagonally in relation to the defender. If this occurs, then it will move the ball closer to them, which will make it easier for them to steal the ball. Remember, the first portion of the self-pass is the bottom of an "L," which will make it a lot easier to dribble the ball past the defender.

Finally, you can perform a shot fake in various ways. You can perform your shot fake using a Cruyff, a step-on step-out, a jump turn, a V pull-back, an outside-of-the-foot cut, or an inside-of-the-foot cut. There is an appropriate time to use each of these in a game. **Being very convincing with a shot fake will allow you to buy that split-second of time when the defender flinches (if they are a few yards from you) or dives in to block the shot (if they are closer to you).** Either scenario will allow you to dribble in the other direction, pass, or find room to shoot. **Furthermore, your shot fake must look exactly like your regular shot!** Ensure that your arms, leg, and head all go up the same way when performing a shot fake and a regular shot.

Develop these Big 3 foot skills to take your game to the next level. Say that you prefer the scissor over the jab step. That is fine, but make sure to practice it nonstop to ensure you are the best at the scissor. Do not waste time and effort trying to learn all the fancy skills that show up on SportsCenter's highlights and in the Top 10 Plays. **In reality, practicing more**

complex moves decreases the amount of time spent on the moves that you know you can successfully use in every game. The "fancy" skills do not produce the same amount of results as the other fundamental (but very efficient) skills. Right now, it is an important time in your soccer career, so you must decide if you want to be a "fancy" player or a player who scores a lot of goals. Choose wisely and choose now, as you will need to take the time to perfect the skills that you will use for years to come.

If you begin to excel with your Big 3 foot skills, and you can now dribble several defenders at once like Lionel Messi can, then it will look fancy. However, if you have not practiced any of these skills before, and your tryout is less than a week away, then I would recommend not working on them yet and instead making sure you practice your strengths leading up to the tryout.

Also, understand that you must read your competition. If you are going against the best player on the team, then you will likely be better off passing the ball. However, if you are going up against someone who is slower than you, then use a skill and your speed to your advantage to reveal how good you are to the coach. But remember that you have to be open to receive a pass, so make quick runs and yell for the ball to ensure you will have possession of it enough times to show off the foot skills that you are comfortable using.

If you are interested in learning how to win in a 1v1, which shot fakes are the best to use, and how to dribble twice as quickly, then grab a copy of the *Understand Soccer* series book, *Soccer Dribbling & Foot Skills*. This book will teach you the keys to becoming the best dribbler in your league and feeling great after every game, knowing that you have several skills you can consistently rely on. Furthermore, as a midfielder or forward, these skills will help you stand out from everyone else at the tryout and make the coach's job easier because it will be obvious that they should select you for the team.

Chapter 11

Receiving a Pass

You can receive the ball with different parts of your foot, but the five general rules to receive a pass (listed in chronological order to ensure ball control and an accurate first touch) are:

1) Plant next to the ball while pointing your foot and hips at your teammate.
2) Toe up, heel down, and ankle locked.
3) Knees slightly bent.
4) Foot slightly off the ground.
5) Typically, use the inside of the foot towards the heel to take an attacking touch.

The form to receive a pass is the same as the first four steps of the form to make a pass. However, to receive a pass, there are a few more things to consider to make sure that you are productive with the ball.

Demand the ball; do not ask for the ball. Yell for the ball; do not call for the ball. These shifts in wording (demand versus ask and yell versus call) do a few excellent things for you, the person that wants to receive a pass or be played a through ball. A through ball is when someone plays the ball in front of you and into space allowing you to run to the ball and continue your forward momentum at full speed.

Demanding the ball lets the person who is passing the ball know that you are very confident. It tells them that you will do something with the ball that is beneficial for your team. Imagine you are in a tryout, and there are two people whom you can pass the ball to. The first person is screaming their head off, demanding the ball. The other person is showing for a pass, using a hand motion to indicate that they want the ball, or meekly asking for the ball. Even if the person yelling for the ball is not quite as open, the player with the ball will consider passing to them first because they can hear that they plan to do something with the ball. Also, demanding/yelling for the ball even if the person with the ball is close to you, ensures that they hear you. Lastly, demanding the ball with confidence gets the coaching staff's attention and reveals that you are a good player.

Often, the person dribbling the ball is far away from you, or they may have a defender or two covering them. Therefore, by demanding and yelling for the ball, you will let them know that you are open to receive the ball. **Many available passes in soccer are not made because the player with the ball did not know that the other player was open.** They have their head down and are looking at the ball to protect the ball from the defender. Therefore, if they do not hear you with their ears, then they are not likely going to see you with their eyes.

Finally, yelling for the ball builds confidence in yourself and increases your ability to help your team achieve its offensive objective of scoring.

Depending on the situation in the tryout, you want to make sure that you check to the ball (go towards the ball) in most instances. More often than not, when you are receiving a pass, you should be checking to the ball to make sure that you successfully receive the ball. Waiting for the ball to travel to you risks a defender intercepting the pass. You definitely do not want to do that when you are making a "through" run and you want the pass played in front of you. In those situations, you want to communicate (e.g., yell/hand motion/or start sprinting in a direction away from the play, but down the field) to them where you are going and let them pass the ball in front of you so that you can take your first touch in stride.

A frustrating thing for a coach at a tryout is when you are passed a good (not a great) pass and you are not able to receive the ball because you are playing lazily. Not checking to the ball tells the coach a lot about the amount of effort you are willing to put forward. You must be active, on your toes, and going to receive the pass. If you do not, it allows the defender to come between you and the ball. This laziness results in an intercepted pass, which makes it very easy for the other team to have a counterattack due to you losing possession during a simple pass.

Before receiving a pass, make sure to scan the field and look behind you. Having a good idea of what you plan to do before you do it will make you a much more effective soccer player and teammate. It does not have to be a 5-10-second scan. It should be just a quick swivel of your head to see if there is pressure, and where some open teammates are so that you can make a sensible pass or dribble into the space after you receive the ball. This is an especially important tip for midfielders or forwards, who are receiving the ball with their back facing the net in which they need to score. A quick look is something that sets college players apart from high school players—and definitely professional players from college players!

These differences are things that coaches and scouts notice at tryouts. An excellent defender, midfielder, or striker will know where teammates and opponents are on the field. Therefore, as they are receiving the pass, they are already thinking about what their next actions in the tryout will be. In soccer and life, if you fail to plan, you plan to fail. **By quickly** scanning behind you, you are already starting to give yourself time to develop a plan of attack. The fast scan will surely help you score more often or let you deliver the pass that will allow your team to score.

Next, when you receive a pass in most game/tryout situations, you still want your hips to be square with your teammate. Though when you are along a sideline this advice may change, being squared with your teammate means that you are pointing your hips at your teammate. When your hips are square with your teammate, you will be more accurate with your first touch than if your hips are not pointing at your teammate. In this instance, you are creating an "L" with your stance by pointing your plant foot at your teammate. The foot that you are receiving the pass with is turned, so you can use the inside of your foot to take your first touch. This form is basically the same as if you were making a pass.

Roughly 95% of your first touches in a tryout should be attacking touches. An attacking touch does not mean you always take a touch toward the other team's goal. An attacking touch simply pushes the ball into space with your first touch to create more room and more time for you to act. An attacking touch is the alternative to taking a touch where the ball stops at your feet. An attacking touch may go towards your opponent's net, towards your own net, or in any direction away from where a defender can reach the ball. In a tryout, you should mostly be taking attacking touches because it allows you, with your first touch, to already have the ball going in the direction that you want to take it.

More often than not, the first attacking touch is into a space on the field to give yourself more time to think, pass, dribble, shoot, or do whatever you need to do with the ball. By taking the first step with your attacking touch, you will have a more accurate first touch. Looking at the picture, Part B is the part of your foot that you would use to take an attacking touch. It is the hardest part of your foot and can be referred to as the "bat."

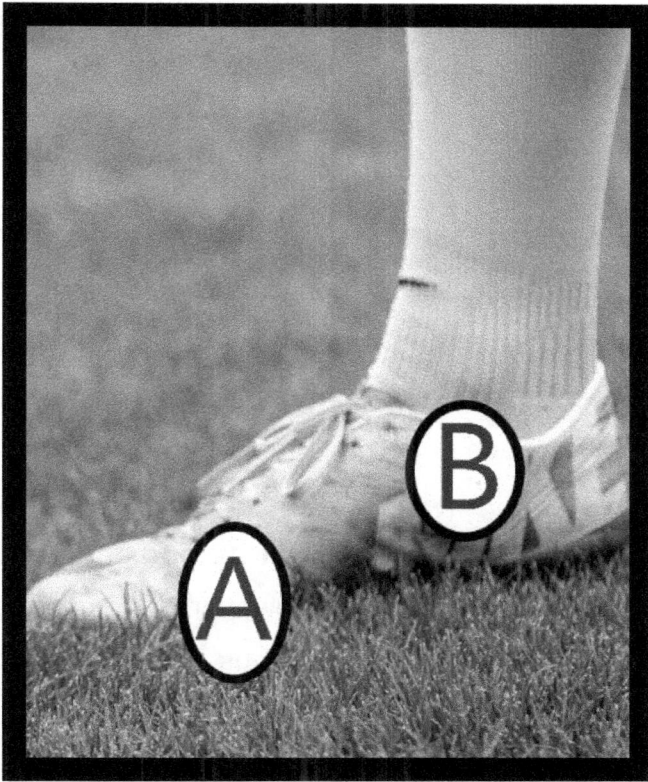

Your attacking touch is not meant to push the ball really far away from you; it is intended for you to take your first step in the direction that you want to go. **For the longest time, I did not realize that an attacking touch is a key to becoming a fast soccer player.** I thought that you had to be a quick runner to be a fast soccer player. In reality, you have to be great with your first attacking touch/step to be a fast soccer player. This one tip alone changed my game overnight. An attacking touch helps your acceleration tremendously because you are already starting to build momentum and speed in the direction that you want to go, which will then enable you to distance yourself from the defender who is marking you.

Occasionally, it will be appropriate to take a touch underneath your body (e.g., a touch that stops at your feet). This touch is necessary when you have too many people around you, and someone could easily cut an attacking touch off and take possession of the ball from you. Only then is it okay to take your first touch underneath your body.

Also, if you receive a difficult pass, then ideally you will still take an attacking first touch. However, it is understandable if you must take a first touch that stops underneath you before you start attacking with the ball. Bad passes are generally played to you in the air. Using the previous picture as reference, Part A would be used to take a touch and settle the ball at your feet. It is the softest portion of your foot, which can be referred to as the "broom."

When you move to receive the pass, what you plan to do next with the ball determines which portion of your foot to use to take an attacking touch. **Ideally, the attacking touch will really be an attacking step.** You push the ball with the same portion of your foot (i.e., the inside of your ankle) that you pass a ball with because it will be locked to push the ball better. However, if you want the ball to stop underneath you, take your first touch with the inside of your foot up towards your toes.

There is space in your shoe between your toes, there is a lot more fabric, and a lot less bone towards your toes. This area of your foot is your "broom" and because your "broom" is not very hard, the ball will stop underneath you. Look at the portion of the foot labeled "A" in the previous image. **Additionally, if you want your first touch to go completely behind you so that you can accelerate away from pressure and into space, then you can take the touch even more softly towards the inside of your foot using your toes (i.e., using the "broom").** Do this more softly than if you wanted to stop the ball underneath you. The softer touch ensures that the ball does not go racing by you. You slow it down a little bit, but do not stop it entirely because you want to be attacking in the space directly behind you.

In conclusion, remember that roughly 95% of your first touches in a tryout should be attacking touches. This tip is the key to increasing your confidence at tryouts because an attacking touch into space gives you more time to think, pass, dribble, lift your head, and shoot. Making enough time for each of these steps will allow you to perform them better and look like a better player to the coaches. To ensure your confidence is high when receiving the ball in a tryout, grab a copy of the *Understand Soccer* series book, *Soccer Passing & Receiving*.

Chapter 12

Outwork Everyone

Tryouts are surely the time to give 100%. If you make the team that you are trying out for, you will receive months and months of quality training that will help you throughout your playing career. Therefore, it is a must that you impress the coaches with your work ethic during the tryout.

Work your butt off in every opportunity. Tryouts are not a time to take it easy and conserve energy. Show the coach you have a terrific fitness and work ethic. Coaches notice effort and even if you make mistakes, coaches understand that you will grow from the mistakes if you continue to work as hard as you can to overcome them.

In order to outwork others, go after the 50/50 balls, help the coach pick up cones, do not stop running when the ball is near you on the field. Though this takes a lot of energy in the moment, you want to walk away from the tryout with your head held high knowing that you gave it your all. Nothing nags you in the back of your mind like living with the regret that you know you could have made the team if you had given it everything. This all out mindset was important for me to use considering my foot skills, shooting ability, defending skills, and speed were not as good as many of the players I was trying out against.

Lastly, be aggressive and use your body. One way to do this and show to the coach you are tough enough for the team is by effectively shielding the ball from other soccer players on the opposing team in the scrimmages. It is crucial that you protect the ball to ensure that you can distribute it to your teammates.

To shield the ball appropriately, consider the following three things:

1) Keep a low center of gravity.
2) Spread your arms.
3) Push the ball away from pressure.

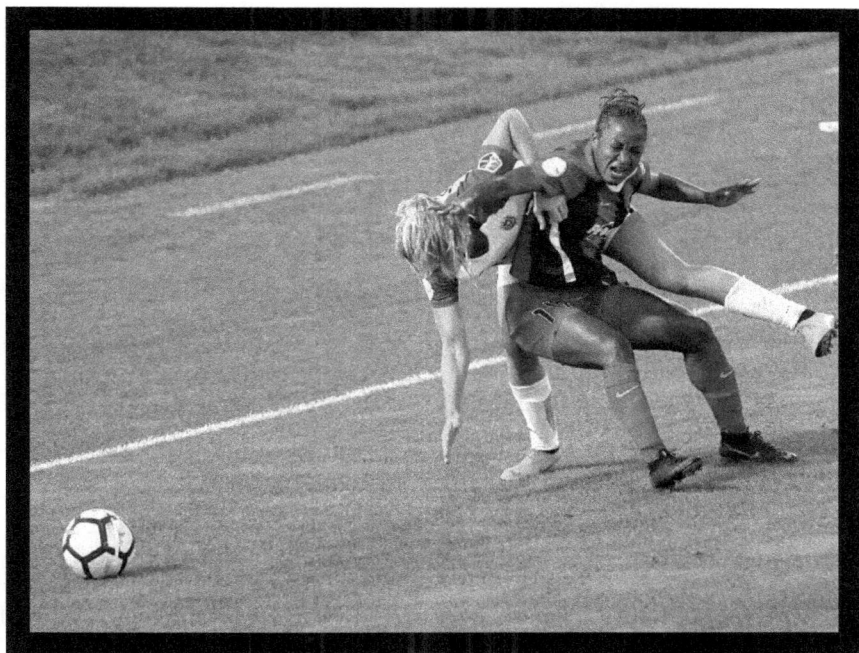

When shielding the ball with an opposing player behind you, it is vital to keep a lower center of gravity than the opponent who is reaching for the ball. A lower center of gravity will give you a solid foundation to make it nearly impossible for the other player to move you and take possession of the ball. Your center of gravity is how high your hips are from the ground, so within reason, bringing your hips down several inches—or even a full foot—will make you are more stable and more difficult to push off the ball. This position is similar to that of a quarter-squat, in which you squat 1/4 of the way down. This position is optimal to shield the ball from the other team.

Keep your arms out. This means extending at both the shoulder and the elbow to make your body and your arms as wide as possible. Although you are often taught from a young age that you are not supposed to keep your elbows or even your arms up, the referees will hardly ever call you out for having your arm raised—especially when you are shielding the ball from a player on the other team. Keeping your arms out and using them as leverage to make it more difficult for the opposition to steal the ball will increase your chance of effectively shielding the ball and passing it to a teammate. Keeping your arms out naturally makes you wider and therefore it will take longer for the opposing player to travel around your body and arms to steal the ball. Even if the opponent does manage to do this, you can take a touch away from them to buy you more time. Use the area on your forearm between your wrist and elbow to make contact. This will provide you with the best advantage, while still putting enough space between the ball and the defender.

When shielding a ball, it is important that you are not afraid to take a touch away from pressure. **A touch away from pressure will help generate some momentum and buy you more time to decide how you will pass the ball to a teammate.** If a player on the other team is coming to your right side behind you, then push the ball more towards the left and vice versa. Having the ball on the side away from the opposition allows you to keep your body entirely between the ball and the other team's player.

Obviously, your size and the size of your opponent does make a difference. If you are a 5'5" soccer player and you are going up against a 6'5" opponent, you will find that their leg length and natural strength will make it difficult for you to shield the ball. **If you are at a significant size disadvantage, avoid situations where you may be required to shield the ball.** This excerpt from the *Understand Soccer* series book, *Soccer Defending*, is critical to outworking the other players on the field.

In summary, the tryout is the place to work the hardest you possibly can. Leave each day of the tryout exhausted to dramatically increase your chance of making the team. Even if your skills do not compare to other players on the field, your work ethic can still be the deciding factor that makes the coach select you.

Chapter 13

Mistakes Are Okay

Steve Corder, a former Division 1 college coach and soccer player at the University of Detroit Mercy, once said something to a group that he was training that left a lasting impression on me. Steve stated, ***"In soccer and in life, you will make hundreds of thousands of mistakes over your lifetime. Once the mistake occurs, it no longer matters that you made the mistake; it only matters how you react to the mistake."***

Most people see mistakes and failures as the same thing. **However, failures are mistakes that have been left uncorrected.** If you make a mistake, then learn from it and correct your actions; this is how you can quickly succeed. Life's greatest lessons are usually learned at the worst times and from the greatest mistakes. In the quote in the previous paragraph, Steve is saying that you cannot get caught up in your past actions. Instead, you must do whatever you can in the present to place yourself in the best situation to succeed in the future. Therefore, if you just made a mistake, then the best thing you can do is take responsibility for it, figure out what happened, learn from it, and then move on.

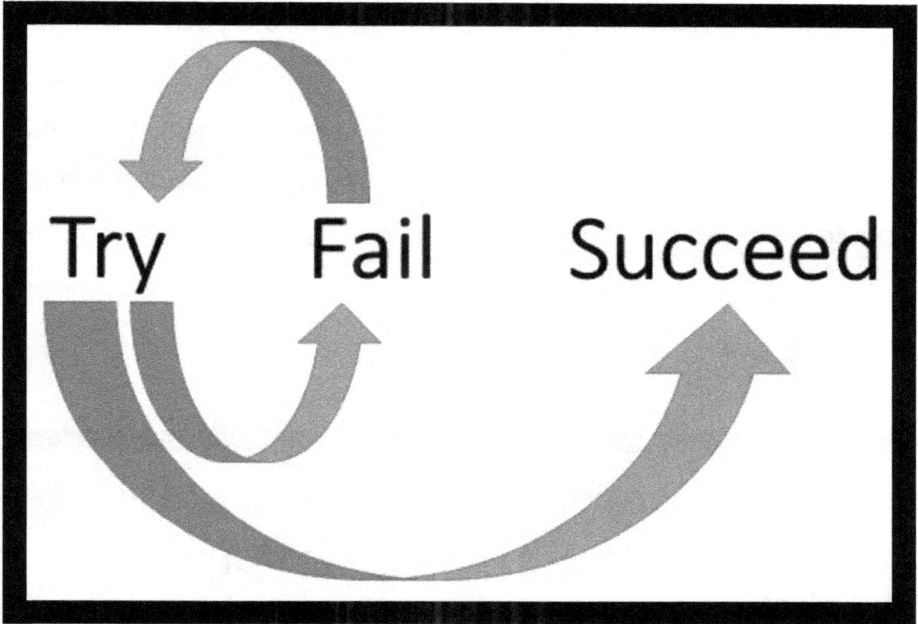

Try   Fail   Succeed

Personally, I suffered for years from the fear of not being perfect. This caused me not to do many things because I was worried about what others would think. Even worse, I was crippled with fear because of my laser-like focus on the mistakes I made. When I did something, I had to check it three times. Then, after reading several books to improve my view of mistakes, I swung too far in the other direction to where I was not concerned *enough* about errors, to the point at which I was not even checking my work at all. This was bad because I mentally became okay with making mistakes, but I was not taking the steps necessary to *learn* from them.

When working on something, check your work just once. Any more than that, and you are likely just wasting time. Not checking your work at all will create sloppy and lazy mistakes. Again, mistakes are great learning tools, but there is a fine line between doing your best in a reasonable period of time but still making a mistake, as opposed to being lazy and sloppy and making *careless* mistakes.

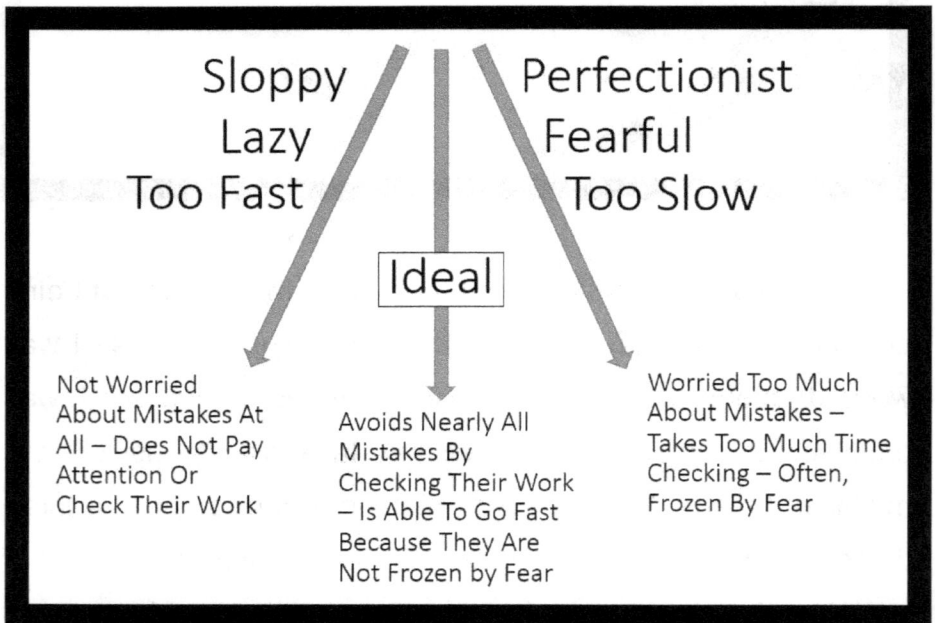

Sloppy Lazy Too Fast	Ideal	Perfectionist Fearful Too Slow
Not Worried About Mistakes At All – Does Not Pay Attention Or Check Their Work	Avoids Nearly All Mistakes By Checking Their Work – Is Able To Go Fast Because They Are Not Frozen by Fear	Worried Too Much About Mistakes – Takes Too Much Time Checking – Often, Frozen By Fear

For example, perhaps the coach at the tryout is demonstrating a dribbling and foot skills drill that you will need to perform. Perfectionists would have anxiety about going through the drill because they might make mistakes. They would want to be the last one in the line and watch the others perform the drill first, so hopefully no one would still be watching if they made a mistake.

On the other hand, sloppy players would go through the drill and make mistakes at seemingly every cone because they did not pay attention as the coach was giving directions.

It is ideal to be the person in the front of the line who is helping the coach demonstrate the drill, actively watching, listening to the coach's directions on what to do at each set of cones, and understanding that they may make a mistake or two on their first lap and/or while helping the coach demonstrate how to perform the drill. But even if this person makes a mistake during the demonstration, they have already done a good portion of the drill and will have learned from their mistakes when going through the drill the second time.

As stated earlier, remember the importance of showing your strengths and hiding your weaknesses as much as possible at a tryout. If dribbling or passing is a major weakness for you, then volunteering to help the coach demonstrate the drill may not be the best option. Instead, you may be good at shooting and want to be the first one in line to help the coach demonstrate the shooting drill instead. Make sure to get in front of the coach as much as possible—especially when you are strong in the area that is being worked on.

In conclusion, avoid lazy mistakes but do not be so worried about being perfect in everything you do. Hustle to win the ball back if you lose it and recover as best you can. Albert Einstein was right when he said, *"Anyone who has never made a mistake has never tried anything new."*

Chapter 14

Bonus Tips

Here are some important miscellaneous tips that will help you make the team:

1) **Get a physical examination, if needed.** Many middle school, junior high school, and high school soccer teams require a doctor's physical examination on file for you to try out. There is not much worse than showing up for the tryout and missing the entire first day because you do not have a physical examination on file with the school.

2) **How much does it cost?** Most teams do not charge you to try out, but there often is a fee to play the entire season with the team. This can be anywhere from a few hundred dollars to a few thousand dollars. Depending on the team you join, and the amount of traveling to tournaments there is, the cost can add up. Take an hour or two several days before the tryout to understand the costs associated with the team, as this may impact your decision to try out.

3) **Bring enough water and sunscreen.** Tryouts often occur in the summer. Being dehydrated will limit your effectiveness, and if you get a sunburn on the first day, it will probably give you

sinus problems, which will make sleeping harder and will definitely impact your performance during the next 1-2 days of the tryout. Therefore, bring more than enough water, and some sunscreen to avoid getting a sunburn.

4) **Make a checklist.** Before you leave the house, make sure you have everything you need including a ball and potentially a snack depending on how long the tryout lasts. Grab the 1-page free checklist at UnderstandSoccer.com/free-printout to make sure you do not forget anything.

5) **Ask questions.** When you do not understand something, be sure to ask for clarification. It may seem awkward to ask for help, but you will look much more awkward if you mess up the drill because you did not understand what was going on!

6) **Warm up before the tryout starts.** Jogging and dynamic stretches are best. Grab a copy of the *Understand Soccer* series book, *Soccer Fitness*, to ensure that you know how to warm up your muscles and fill your joints with synovial fluids.

7) **Stretch and ice.** Although stretching after the tryout is not the most glamourous thing; it will help your recovery and keep you fresher than your competition. This is easy to do for 10 minutes at the conclusion of each day of tryouts—but it is also just as easy to forget!

8) **Do not be silly.** You can be a great soccer player but not make the team or even get kicked off the team. In fact, when I was in high school, there was a player that swore at the wrong moment and was cut from the team because of it. Does this seem a bit ridiculous? Yes. But, does it happen? Yes.

9) **Be competitive and attempt to win everything during the tryout.** Remember that at the end of the day, the coach needs winners on their team. Be competitive and work hard to come out on top. Coaches are competitive and want to win. They want their players to have the same drive, too.

10) **Pick the team that will help you develop the most.** Chris Klein, former U.S. Men's National Team player, MLS star, and Senior Director at the LA Galaxy Academy, says, *"My advice for youth players is to go to a club program where you think you can develop the most. Find a positive environment where you can develop your skills."* Therefore, though winning is important, becoming a better soccer player yourself is even more important. If you make multiple teams, consider everything and heavily weigh which club you will be better able to develop as a soccer player.

11) **Have fun!** You got this! This is an opportunity for you to show your stuff and enjoy the journey. Tryouts can be scary—

but only if you view them as such. If you view them as "exciting" instead, you will have more energy and perform better on the day of the tryout. Have fun while playing and remember why you are trying out—because you love this beautiful sport!

YouTube: If you would like to see a video on tips for tryouts, then consider watching the *Understand Soccer* YouTube video: *Soccer Tryout Tips*.

Afterword

Congrats! Because you read this book, you gained a ton of knowledge about how to do well in your tryout(s). Implement the tips mentioned to double or even triple your chances of making the team.

Even more importantly, in addition to the knowledge you have gained, you have also increased your confidence. This is huge! Just by reading this book and doing what it mentions, you are giving yourself a massive advantage over your competitors. Knowing that you already have these advantages as you go into the tryout will boost your confidence, reduce your nervousness, and increase your excitement about the tryout. As a friend, I know you have got this tryout. You are awesome!

By reading this book, you have shown that you care a lot about making the team, and I applaud you for it. So many other players are not willing to take just a few hours to learn the tools and information that can make tryouts and all other areas of their soccer career much easier and twice as fun. But you just did! Great job!

Excitingly, that is what a book can do. A book takes a person's decades of experiences—all their highs, lows, and knowledge—and then condenses that information into something that you can read in a few hours. Think about it—you just spent a few hours learning what took me an entire career to learn! Because of that, I know you will have a great tryout.

Best of luck at your tryout and be sure to let me know how it went!

If the tips you read in this book helped you gain confidence before a tryout or helped you make the team, please leave a positive review on Amazon.com to let me know!

WAIT!

Wouldn't it be nice to have the steps in this book on an easy one-page checklist for you to make preparing and succeeding in your tryouts even easier? Well, here is your chance!

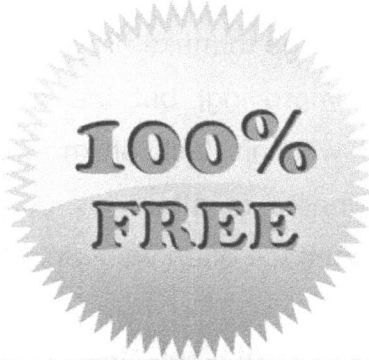

UNDERSTANDSOCCER.COM - TRYOUT CHECKLIST

✔ **Before Tryouts Start**
- Avoid working out at least two days prior to the start of tryouts.
- Eat a nutritious meal. (I.e. chicken, a fruit, a vegetable, and a grain/carb.)
- Have all your gear? (Boil cleats, shin guards, socks, etc.)
- Wear the same bright color each day to stand out.
- Bring your medical physical, if needed.
- Apply sunscreen if it is a sunny day.
- Bring snacks like a banana or apple if the tryout is several hours.
- Drink a 16 oz. water bottle to make sure that you are hydrated.
- 30 mins prior to start, drink a pre-workout like: Pure Pump
      Watermelon Naked Energy   Garden of Life Energy + Focus
- Get to the field early (at least 30 mins).
- Remember, the feelings you have right now are feelings of excitement.
- Warm up for at least 10 minutes before the actual tryouts start.

✔ **During Tryouts**
- Make a great first impression - Shake the coach's hand and introduce yourself.
- Make eye contact, smile, and stand up straight.
- Tryout in the position you want to play.
- Show off you strengths.
- Communicate & direct other people what to do in scrimmages.
- If a coach gives you feedback, implement it immediately.
- Make sure at least 95% of your first touches are attacking touches.
- Outwork others. Hustle, hustle, hustle!
- If you make a mistake, don't sweat it. Recover from it as best you can.
- Drink a 16 oz. bottle of water for every hour of tryouts.

✔ **After Tryouts**
- Thank the coach & give him or her another strong handshake.
- Stretch.
- Ice any body parts that hurt once you get home.
- Drink a 16 oz. water bottle to help with recovery.
- Take a post workout whey protein supplement or drink some milk.

©Understand, LLC

Go to this Link for an **Instant** One-Page Printout:
UnderstandSoccer.com/free-printout

This FREE checklist is simply a "Thank You" for purchasing this book. This one-page checklist will ensure that the knowledge you obtain from this book helps you make the team.

About the Author

There he was—a soccer player who had difficulties scoring. He wanted to be the best on the field but lacked the confidence and knowledge to make his goal a reality. Every day, he dreamed about improving, but the average coaching he received, combined with his lack of knowledge, only left him feeling alone and unable to attain his goal. He was a quiet player, and his performance often went unnoticed.

This all changed after his junior year on the varsity soccer team of one of the largest high schools in the state. During the team and parent banquet at the end of the season, his coach decided to say something nice about each player. When it was his turn to receive praise, the only thing that could be said was that he had scored two goals that season—even though they were against a lousy team, so they didn't really count. It was a very painful statement that after the 20+ game season, all that could be said of his efforts were two goals that didn't count. One of his greatest fears came true; he was called out in front of his family and friends.

Since that moment, he was forever changed. He got serious. With a new soccer mentor, he focused on training to obtain the necessary skills, build his confidence, and become the goal-scorer that he'd always dreamed of being. The next season, after just a few months, he found himself moved up to the starting position of center midfielder and scored his first goal of the 26-game season in only the third game.

He continued with additional training led by a proven goal-scorer to build his knowledge. Fast-forward to the present day, and, as a result of the work he put in, and his focus on the necessary skills, he figured out how to become a goal-scorer who averages about two goals and an assist per game—all because he increased his understanding of how to play soccer. With the help of a soccer mentor, he took his game from being a bench-warmer who got called out in front of everybody to becoming the most confident player on the field.

Currently, he is a soccer trainer in Michigan, working for Next Level Training. He advanced through their rigorous program as a soccer player and was hired as a trainer. This program has allowed him to guide world-class soccer players for over a decade. He trains soccer players in formats ranging from one-hour classes to weeklong camps, and he instructs classes of all sizes, from groups of 30 soccer players all the way down to working one-on-one with individuals who want to play for the United States National Team.

If you enjoyed this book, then please leave a review.

Additional Books by Dylan Joseph Available on Amazon:

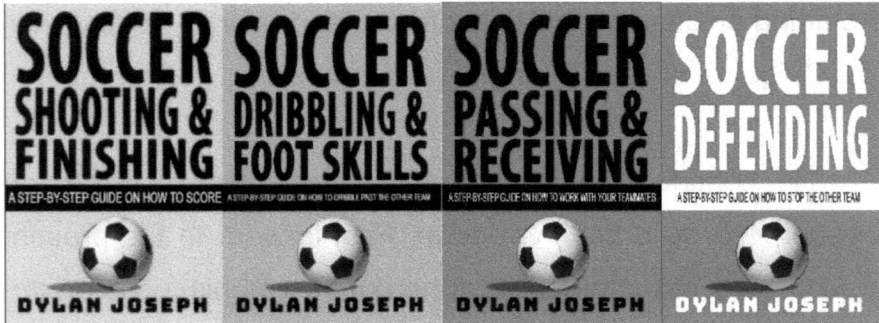

Soccer Shooting & Finishing: A Step-by-Step Guide on How to Score

Soccer Dribbling & Foot Skills: A Step-by-Step Guide on How to Dribble Past the Other Team

Soccer Passing & Receiving: A Step-by-Step Guide on How to Work with Your Teammates

Soccer Defending: A Step-by-Step Guide on How to Stop the Other Team

Free Book!

How would you like to get a book of your choosing in the *Understand Soccer* series for free?

Join the Soccer Squad Book Team today and receive your next book (and potentially future books) for FREE.

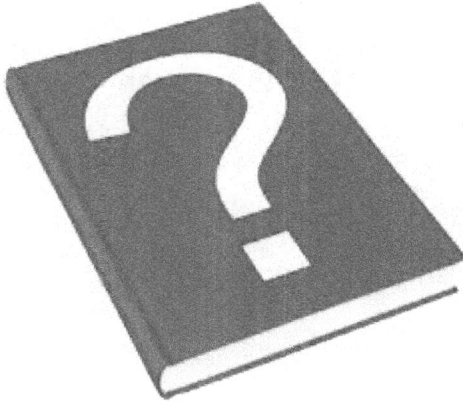

Signing up is easy and does not cost anything.

Check out this website for more information:

UnderstandSoccer.com/soccer-squad-book-team

Thank You for Reading!

Dear Reader,

I hope you enjoyed and learned from **Soccer Tryouts**. I truly enjoyed writing these steps and tips to ensure you can easily make the team.

As an author, I love feedback. Candidly, you are the reason that I wrote this book and plan to write more. Therefore, tell me what you liked, what you loved, and what can be improved. I'd love to hear from you. Visit UnderstandSoccer.com and scroll to the bottom of the homepage to leave me a message in the contact section or email me at:

Dylan@UnderstandSoccer.com

Finally, I need to ask a favor. **I'd love and truly appreciate a review.**

As you likely know, reviews are a key part of my process to see whether you, the reader, enjoyed my book. The reviews allow me to write more books. You have the power to help make or break my book. Please take the 2 minutes to leave a review on Amazon.com at: https://www.amazon.com/gp/product-review/1949511251.

In gratitude,

Dylan Joseph

Glossary

50-50 - When a ball is passed into pressure or cleared up the field and your teammate and a player on the opposing team each have an equal (50%) chance of taking possession of the soccer ball.

Additives/Fillers - A substance, often artificial, added to food in small quantities to improve it, preserve it, or to add to its weight so it seems like you are getting more for your money.

Adrenaline - Released by your body to increase rate of blood circulation, breathing, and metabolism to prepare muscles for use.

Antioxidants - A substance that inhibits damaging oxidation in the body.

Attacking Touch - Pushing the ball into space with your first touch, which is the opposite of taking a touch where the ball stops underneath you (i.e., at your feet).

Bat - The bone (i.e., hardest portion) of your foot.

Blood Sugar - The concentration of glucose in the blood.

Broom - In this book, it is the area on your foot towards your toes. There is space in your shoe between your toes where there is a lot more fabric and a lot less bone, which makes it a soft area on your foot, similar to the softness of a broom.

Caffeine - A central nervous system stimulant that gives you energy and mental focus.

Carbohydrates - Sugars, starch, and cellulose that typically can be broken down to release energy in the human body.

Championship - A match to determine the champion in the league. This is usually the final game of the season.

Comfort Zone - A psychological state where things feel familiar to a person and they are at ease and in control of their environment while experiencing low levels of anxiety and stress.

Creatine - A compound formed in protein metabolism. It is involved in the supply of energy for muscular contraction and aids in recovery after a workout. It can be made in the liver, kidney, and pancreas using the three amino acids Arginine, Glycine, and Methionine.

Cruyff - Cut the ball, but leave yourself between the defender and the ball. In essence, you are cutting the ball behind your plant leg.

Cut - This is performed with the inside of your foot. The leg that is cutting the ball must step entirely past the ball. Then, allow the ball to hit that leg/foot, which effectively stops the ball. Having the ball stop next to your foot enables the ball to be pushed in a different direction quickly. Additionally, you may cut the ball so that it is immediately moving in the direction that you want to go.

Delayed Onset Muscle Soreness ("DOMS") - The pain and stiffness felt in muscles several hours to several days after strenuous exercise. The soreness is felt most strongly 24 to 72 hours after the exercise.

Dextrose - A simple sugar that digests very quickly and acts as blood sugar in the body.

Fat - Along with proteins and carbohydrates, this is one of the three nutrients used as energy sources by the body. This is how the body stores a majority of its energy.

Gluten - A substance present in many grains, especially wheat, that is responsible for the elastic texture of dough. It can damage the gut wall, and may cause nutrient deficiencies, anemia, and digestive issues.

Glycogen - Carbohydrates stored in bodily tissues ready to be used during exercise.

Greek Yogurt - Has more protein and less sugar than regular yogurt.

Growth Mindset - Believing your basic qualities of intelligence, talent, humor, athletic ability, etc. are abilities you have developed over time using knowledge and hard work.

Ingredients - Any of the foods or substances that are combined to make a particular dish.

Jab Step (i.e., "Feint," "Body Feint," "Fake," "Fake and Take," or "Shoulder Drop") - When you pretend to push the ball in one direction, but purposely miss, then plant with the foot that you missed the ball with to push the ball in the other direction.

Jitters - Feelings of nervousness.

Jump Turn - Instead of pulling the ball back with the bottom of your foot, as you would do in the V pull back, stop the ball with the bottom of your foot as you jump past the ball, landing with both feet at the same time on the other side of the ball. Landing with both feet at the same time on the other side of the ball allows you to explode away in the direction from which you came.

Junior Varsity - A team representing a high school or college at the level below varsity.

Medical Physical - Where a medical practitioner performs a physical examination on you for any possible signs or symptoms of a medical condition.

Military Method of Sleeping - Relax your face, including your tongue. Drop your shoulders to release the tension and let your hands drop to the side of your body while lying on your back. Exhale from your chest. Relax your legs, thighs, and calves. Clear your mind for 10 seconds by imagining nothing. Then, try mentally saying the words "don't think" over and over. Within a minute, you should fall asleep!

Minerals - A naturally occurring, inorganic solid substance such as calcium, iron, potassium, sodium, or zinc, that is essential to the nutrition of humans.

National Collegiate Athletic Association ("NCAA") - A nonprofit organization that regulates student athletes from 1,268 North American institutions and conferences.

Nutrition - A substance that provides nourishment essential for growth and the maintenance of life.

Nutrition - Eating the food necessary for health and growth.

Ounce - A unit of weight representing one-sixteenth of a pound (approximately 28 grams).

Perfectionist - A person who often uses wanting to be perfect as an excuse for not getting started.

Phytonutrients - Helps prevent disease and keep your body working properly. The six major phytonutrients are carotenoids, ellagic acid, flavonoids, resveratrol, glucosinolates, and phytoestrogens.

Pre-Workout Supplement - It contains ingredients that are intended to give a sudden boost of energy. These supplements are over the counter and are used by mainly athletes to help aid in performance.

Protein - Large molecules composed of one or more long chains of amino acids and are essential structural components of body tissues such as muscle, hair, collagen, etc.

Psychology - The scientific study of the mind and behavior.

Scissor - When the foot closest to the ball goes around the ball as you are attacking in a game. Emphasize turning your hips to fake the defender. To easily turn your hips, plant past the ball with your foot that is not going around the ball so that you can use the momentum of the moving ball to your advantage.

Self-Pass (i.e., "L," "Iniesta," or "La Croqueta") - Passing the ball from one foot to the other while running. Imagine you are doing a roll, but without your foot going on top of the ball. Instead, it is an inside of the foot pass from one foot and an inside of the foot push up the field with the other foot.

Shot Fake - Faking a shot. Make sure your form looks the same as when you shoot, including: 1) Looking at the goal before you do a shot fake 2) Arms out 3) Raise your shooting leg high enough behind your body, so it looks like you are going to shoot.

Shot Fake - Faking a shot. Make sure your form looks the same as when you shoot, including: 1) Looking at the goal before you do a shot fake 2) Arms out 3) Raise your shooting leg high enough behind your body, so it looks like you are going to shoot.

Slouching - Standing or sitting in a lazy, drooping way.

Small-Sided Scrimmage - These often do not simulate a full game. Rather, they simulate situations that players may encounter during an actual game. Full teams or sides do not compete against each other and every position is not covered. Instead, players are matched up one-on-one, two-on-two, etc.

Sociolinguistics - The descriptive study of the effect of any and all aspects of society, including cultural norms, expectations, and context, on the way language is used, and society's effect on language.

Step-On Step-Out - In order to change direction, step on the ball with the bottom of your foot. Then, with the same foot that stepped on the ball, take another step to plant to the side of the ball, so that your other leg can come through and push the ball in a different direction.

Step-Over - When you are next to the ball and you have your furthest leg from the ball step over the ball, so your entire body turns as if you are going in a completely different direction. The step over is best used along a sideline.

Tryouts - A test of the potential of someone in the context of attempting to make a soccer team.

V Pull Back - Pull the ball backward using the bottom of your foot. Then, use your other leg to push the ball and accelerate forward in the other direction, hence the "V" in the V pull back.

Varsity - The main team representing a high school or college.

Vitamins - Group of organic compounds which are essential for normal growth and nutrition and are required in small quantities in the diet because they cannot be created by the body. Examples include A, C, D, E, and K, choline, and the B vitamins (thiamin, riboflavin, niacin, pantothenic acid, biotin, vitamin B6, vitamin B12, and folate/folic acid).

Whey Protein - Protein contained in the watery portion of milk that separates from the curds when making cheese. Whey protein is commonly used for improving athletic performance and increasing strength. Whey protein concentrate has more fat and lactose that Whey protein isolate. Whey protein concentrate can lead to upset stomachs and flatulence in some consumers.

Acknowledgments

I would like to thank you, the reader. I am grateful to provide you value and to help you on your journey of becoming a more confident soccer player, coach, or parent. I am happy to serve you and thank you for the opportunity to do so. Also, I would like to recognize people that have made a difference and have paved the way for me to share this book with you:

I want to thank the grammar editor Abbey Decker. Her terrific understanding of the complexities of the English language ensured that the wording needed to convey the messages was appropriate and she provided countless grammatical improvements.

Additionally, I would like to thank the content editors Kevin Solorio, Toni Sinistaj, and Youssef Hodroj. They reviewed this book for areas that could be improved and additional insights to share. Without their input, this book would not be the high-quality reading material you have come to expect in the *Understand Soccer* series.

Many thanks,

Dylan Joseph